MILADY'S AESTHETICIAN SERIES: MEDISPA DICTIONARY

Pamela Hill, R.N.

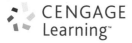

CENGAGE
Learning™

Australia • Brazil • Japan • Korea • Mexico • Singapore • Spain • United Kingdom • United States

CENGAGE
Learning™

Milady's Aesthetician Series: Medispa Dictionary
Pamela Hill, R.N.

President, Milady: Dawn Gerrain

Publisher: Erin O'Connor

Acquisitions Editor: Martine Edwards

Senior Product Manager: Phil Mandl

Editorial Assistant: Elizabeth Edwards

Director of Beauty Industry Relations: Sandra Bruce

Senior Marketing Manager: Gerald McAvey

Production Director: Wendy Troeger

Senior Art Director: Benj Gleeksman

For product information and technology assistance, contact us at **Cengage Learning Customer & Sales Support, 1-800-354-9706**

For permission to use material from this text or product, submit all requests online at **cengage.com/permissions**
Further permissions questions can be emailed to **permissionrequest@cengage.com**

Library of Congress Control Number: 2010940890

ISBN-13: 978-1-4390-6028-5

ISBN-10: 1-4390-6028-2

Milady
5 Maxwell Drive
Clifton Park, NY 12065-2919
USA

Cengage Learning is a leading provider of customized learning solutions with office locations around the globe, including Singapore, the United Kingdom, Australia, Mexico, Brazil, and Japan. Locate your local office at: **international. cengage.com/region**

Cengage Learning products are represented in Canada by Nelson Education, Ltd.

For your lifelong learning solutions, visit **milady.cengage.com**
Visit our corporate website at **www.cengage.com**

Notice to the Reader
Publisher does not warrant or guarantee any of the products described herein or perform any independent analysis in connection with any of the product information contained herein. Publisher does not assume, and expressly disclaims, any obligation to obtain and include information other than that provided to it by the manufacturer. The reader is expressly warned to consider and adopt all safety precautions that might be indicated by the activities described herein and to avoid all potential hazards. By following the instructions contained herein, the reader willingly assumes all risks in connection with such instructions. The publisher makes no representations or warranties of any kind, including but not limited to, the warranties of fitness for particular purpose or merchantability, nor are any such representations implied with respect to the material set forth herein, and the publisher takes no responsibility with respect to such material. The publisher shall not be liable for any special, consequential, or exemplary damages resulting, in whole or part, from the readers' use of, or reliance upon, this material.

Printed in the United States of America
1 2 3 4 5 6 7 12 11 10

BRIEF CONTENTS

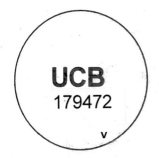

CONTENTS

ABOUT THE AUTHOR

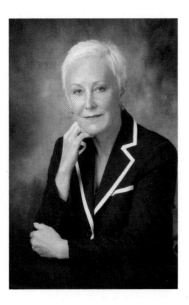

Pamela Hill, R.N., CEO, received her diploma from Presbyterian/St. Luke's Hospital and Colorado Women's College. She followed through to practice as a registered nurse for more than 30 years, with her initial emphasis in cardiac surgery and then in cosmetic surgery and medical skin care. In 1992, Ms. Hill founded Facial Aesthetics, a network of medical skin care clinics in association with John A. Grossman, M.D. Since then, Ms. Hill has been an industry pioneer in the growth and development of the medical spa industry. As the president and chief executive officer of Facial Aesthetics, Ms. Hill has been a proactive member and pioneer in the evolution of the medical spa model and the integration and union of cosmeceuticals and nonsurgical skin care. In addition to her leadership in the medical spa industry, she has also been actively engaged in the research and development of the successful Pamela Hill Skin Care product line.

Ms. Hill has devoted her passion for nonmedical skin care to the instruction of a higher level of education and skill for those aspiring to be the aestheticians of tomorrow.

ACKNOWLEDGMENTS

As with all of my books, the *Medispa Dictionary* has been the effort of many people. But there is no one more important to thank than the staff at Milady, especially Martine Edwards. Martine has always been there, encouraging me even though I might be tired and sometimes a little weary. The reviewers have also been an important aspect of this book, helping us to understand what additional words were needed, which ones could be left out of the text, and where definitions needed improvement. The reviewers are always an important part of the process, and without them, a book such as this would not come to life.

Finally, and as always, a big thank you to my husband John, who gives up time with me so that I can write and share my knowledge.

PREFACE

L ike many other industries, the realm of aesthetics has its own vernacular–that is, its own vocabulary specific to the conditions and treatments performed in a spa environment. Certain words are common and easily learned. Others are not so easy. Treatments and conditions have names you will use every day and need little explanation. However, once you peel back the layers of the proverbial onion, you will discover that there are some terms of this vernacular that you will encounter which you will need to learn.

This is especially true for those of you who choose to embark on a medical aesthetics career. There is no license that defines a medical aesthetician. Rather, it is the courses that begin to prepare an individual for this category and are defined as "master" or "advanced" which qualify an aesthetician to work in a medical environment (such as a dermatologist's or plastic surgeon's office). These courses often deal with microdermabrasion, peels, and education on lasers and injectables. While all of this information is important, one component is left out: the ability to understand and speak medical jargon.

A "medical" aesthetician can be found nearly everywhere these days, from a day spa that injects Botox to any medical office that is offering skin care services. It is a broad term that speaks to the advanced procedures that aestheticians, nurses, and nurse practitioners are providing. But it is competitive out there, and to get a job as a medical aesthetician, one must be qualified. The ability to talk with the physician and nurses in the language they understand gives the aesthetician a competitive edge. Further, it helps the aesthetician to integrate into the medical practice with greater ease. Reading the chart is easier when the aesthetician understands the medical terms written on it. Nothing could be more important. Comprehending the full extent of the client's care only helps the aesthetician to integrate into the medical team. This book is designed with skin care, plastic surgery, and dermatology in mind. The words and terms contained within these pages will be important to understand as you embark on a career in the medical world.

MILADY'S AESTHETICIAN SERIES: MEDISPA DICTIONARY

Successful Communication in the Medispa

Working in the medical spa setting can be challenging. One of the first challenges is getting to know and understand your place in the hierarchy that exists in a medical setting or medical spa. Once you understand your place within the office, there are your contributions to the clinic and the care of the client to consider. The relationships that you build will be, in large part, based on your communication skills. In aesthetics, the degree to which we can or cannot communicate in a medical spa can have far-reaching implications. These implications will extend to the client's well-being, your livelihood, and the overall success of the business. Whether the communication is with the physician, the nurse, the client, or the clinic manager, communication is going to play a part in your success.

In the clinical environment, there exists a special type of vernacular which medical professionals use to communicate—it is called medical terminology. Why a special vernacular, you might ask? Well, to make it simple, it is used to create a universal language of health so that health-related professionals can communicate with one another, regardless of boundaries. The same holds true of aesthetics: we use words to communicate with other aestheticians. These words may define things pertaining to the skin, such as comedones, or refer to equipment, like a maglite.

Every part of our bodies—our senses, our mouths, and our gestures—is engaged in a perpetual transmission of verbal and nonverbal codes from which we send and receive information, assign value levels, and retain (or discard). In similar situations, different people will assign different levels of importance to the same piece of information. In the medical setting, this level of importance is critical in the care of the client; this is why medical vernacular is so important. For example, a physician will define a cut as a laceration. He or she may further define that laceration as epidermal, dermal, or subdermal. Understanding these words and their definitions is critical for the aesthetician who expects to understand the medical environment and to be successful in it.

Types of Communication

Though this book is primarily meant to provide a useful reference on medical terminology and how to use it, there are several types of communication that the successful aesthetician will be familiar with, including interpersonal, verbal, and nonverbal.

Interpersonal Communication

Interpersonal communication, also called dyadic communication, involves communication between one person and another. This type of communication usually involves listening, dialogue exchange, summarizing, paraphrasing, and gesturing. This is typically the kind of communication that is done with colleagues and clients. Interpersonal communication can be conducted between as few as two people, and up to many thousands. Another example of interpersonal communication is found in a classroom. Most often, we use interpersonal communication to communicate with one another. Usually, we are engaged in conversations with no more than a handful of people who are sharing a physical space. Obviously, this is true of the consultation or treatment of a client or with the medical professionals with whom you work.

Verbal Communication

Most often, we use words and language to send information. When a potential sender has a thought or an idea, the verbal communication begins. In order for the receiver to understand the message, it needs to be encoded. Encoding is a cognitive process by which the sender organizes ideas into symbols and vernacular. Those who are adept at verbal communication will take steps to ensure the intended recipient understands the message. To accomplish this, words, actions, and tone are considered and chosen *with the recipient in mind*. The message is decoded and, ideally, received. Verbal communication also involves the use of inflection and volume to send a message. If a person is talking in loud tones, it conveys a different meaning than if the person speaks in a low, monotone fashion, for example.

Nonverbal Communication

Nonverbal communication is the process of sending a message without a verbal cue. While nonverbal communication is usually perceived as "no," it can sometimes mean "yes." The most common non-verbal communication is facial expressions. Remember that old expression "The eyes are the window to the soul"? Your eyes are the most powerful non-verbal communicator. Your eyes can tell others what you are thinking—if you believe in yourself or if you believe the product you recommend has value. Hand gestures, body movements, touch, and personal space also play a role in nonverbal communication. Sometimes silence itself can convey a message. If you are talking during a class and your instructor stops talking and stares at you, you easily ascertain the need to pay attention.

Communication in the Consultation

Membership in the medical and allied medical fields can be complicated in its multifactorial and multifunctional capacities. Knowing which skills to employ at what moment or in synch with other skills you have will require you to engage in a delicate dance between form and function with the appearance of ease and professionalism. This may actually take some time, maybe years to perfect. In fact, there are some schools of thought that say a person will not remember information until the concept is repeated eight times.[1]

Having the knowledge is only one aspect of success in the medical aesthetics industry. Your successes are often driven by the impressions people have of you and the aesthetic industry. We are in an image business. The first impression a new patient will have of your office and your expertise is based in part on the cleanliness of the office, the knowledge and friendliness of the staff, and last but certainly not least, your appearance. All of these aspects communicate something about you. Be sure what you are communicating is the message you want to be sending.

During the consultation, a patient's ability to listen and hear your information is affected by how comfortable they feel. That *comfort zone* includes how "medical" the room appears (this can be intimidating), the seating arrangement, and your professionalism. Professionalism relates to your appearance, knowledge, and command of the language.

Mastering the skills of friendliness, cleanliness, comfort, professionalism, and communication can all impact the patient's first and lasting impressions.

Furthermore, the perception the patient has of you is one that extends to your physician, your colleagues, and the rest of the staff at the spa. The impression the patient has of you and the facility will determine trust, which is the foundation of any relationship.

Relationships are built on trust. In the medical spa, this is best achieved through the position of education. As we begin to educate our clients rather than sell, our client relationships begin to solidify. Sharing information and educating clients through our medical knowledge and medical vernacular demonstrate skills that evolve into trust. Communication is a large part of the relationship.

Communication with the Medical Staff

Communication with the medical staff typically surrounds the status of a client. Your ability to evaluate and quickly communicate a client's status is important to the medical staff and to the quality of care the client will receive. Further, your ability to use the proper medical vernacular will allow the client's condition, progress, and status to be communicated in a manner that allows the medical professional to understand exactly what you are trying to say. This use of the medical vernacular allows for quick easy diagnosis and treatment of the client. Discussing the client using the medical vernacular also puts you in a more professional light. It will, in part, improve your relationships within the facility as the medical professionals will begin to trust your knowledge and, finally, your abilities.

Conclusion

Not enough can be said about finding the vernacular that is important in your aesthetics sector and using it appropriately. Above all, we must communicate well in order to be successful in our chosen career. Communication with colleagues in an appropriate and professional manner furthers your standing in the business community. Moreover, it helps you to educate and build relationships with clients.

Chapter Reference

1. Lavington, C. (1997). *You've only got three seconds.* New York: Broadway Books.

CHAPTER 2

The Importance of Understanding Anatomy and Physiology

All of us would like to know more about our bodies; we want and need to understand what makes the inner parts of us work. For example, babies are mesmerized by simply looking at their toes, while adults worry and wonder about a shortness of breath. *Anatomy and physiology* is a subset of biology; it is the study of the human body and how it is put together.

Anatomy is the study of the structures themselves, while **physiology** is the science of the bodily functions. In reality, they are interrelated. Anatomy cannot happen without physiology and vice versa. When we look at and study the muscles and muscle names or bones and bone names we are discussing *gross anatomy*. On the other hand, if we are involving a microscope and looking at the cellular structure of the muscles or bones, this is called *microscopic anatomy*.

> **Did you know?**
>
> The word **anatomy** means to cut apart.
>
> **Ana** is Greek for part and **tomy** is Greek for cut.

Physiology is the study of how the parts of the body—the anatomy—functions. Physiology has many subsections, such as *endrocrine physiology* or *cardiac physiology*. The parts of the body are always related and form a planned entity. Each "part" is necessary to make the entire unit work as a well-oiled machine.

For example, the bones create the skeleton that makes our body stable, but the muscles around the bones make the bones function. Each system (Figure 2–1) has its purpose and its own anatomy and physiology, but it is all intertwined to make the entire unit work together to create the human body.

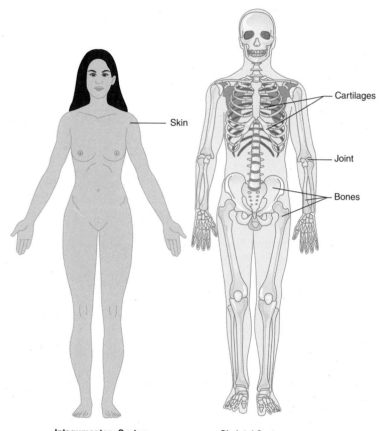

Integumentary System
Commonly known as the skin. It helps to control the temperature of the body and protects the body from the outside environment by making us aware of pain, for example.

Skeletal System
Commonly known for the bones but also includes the cartilages, ligaments, and joints. The skeletal system helps to provide support and protection to internal organs.

Figure 2–1 Each system within the body has its purpose and its own anatomy and physiology, but it is all intertwined to make the entire unit work together to create the human body. © Milady, a part of Cengage Learning

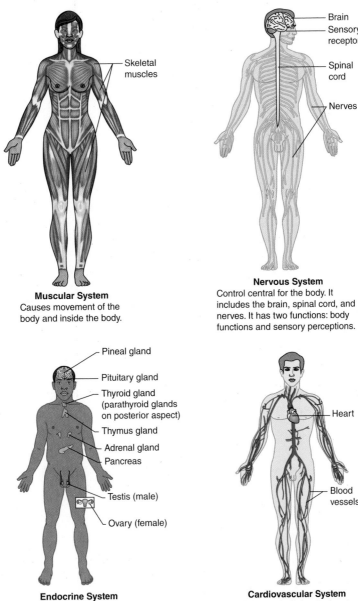

Muscular System
Causes movement of the
body and inside the body.

Skeletal
muscles

Nervous System
Control central for the body. It
includes the brain, spinal cord, and
nerves. It has two functions: body
functions and sensory perceptions.

Brain
Sensory
receptor
Spinal
cord
Nerves

Endocrine System
Controls the body's activities slowly
through the glands that are placed
specifically about the body.

Pineal gland
Pituitary gland
Thyroid gland
(parathyroid glands
on posterior aspect)
Thymus gland
Adrenal gland
Pancreas
Testis (male)
Ovary (female)

Cardiovascular System
This system includes the heart
and the blood vessels with blood
as the fluid that transports oxygen
and nutrients to the cells.

Heart
Blood
vessels

Figure 2–1 (continued)

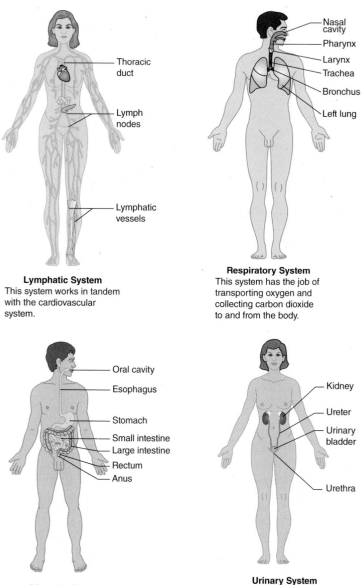

Lymphatic System
This system works in tandem with the cardiovascular system.

Respiratory System
This system has the job of transporting oxygen and collecting carbon dioxide to and from the body.

Digestive System
Carries the food from the mouth through the system and out the anus for waste. It uses the blood to disperse nutrients to the body.

Urinary System
Disposes of liquid waste from the body through the kidneys, ureters, and bladder. Electrolyte balance is also an important part of this system's responsibility.

Figure 2–1 (continued)

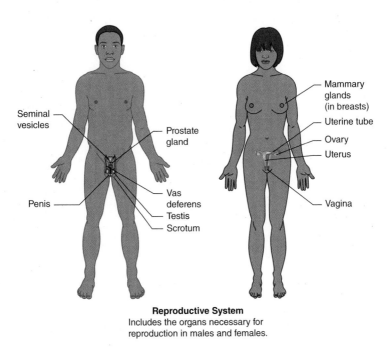

Reproductive System
Includes the organs necessary for
reproduction in males and females.

Figure 2–1 (continued)

As an aesthetician working in the plastic surgery, dermatology, or another special sector of medicine, it is important to understand the anatomy and physiology of the human body so that you can better care for your client. This knowledge helps us to understand why clients take certain medications or have certain skin conditions or diseases that we need to be aware of in our treatments.

An Overview of the Human Body

The human body is complex and made up of many different cell types. One could view the body as a *ladder* that begins at the chemical level, which involves atoms that form molecules. The molecules, depending on their type, eventually form together to create cells (Figure 2–2). The cells will vary in size and shape depending on their function within the body. All living matter is made up of cells. The main parts of the cell are the nucleus, the cytoplasm, and the cell membrane (Figure 2–3). Moving up the ladder within the structure of the human body, the next level is the tissues, which are formed based on the similar cells available. There are four basic tissue types within the body: epithelial, connective, muscular, and neural (Figure 2–4). Each cell

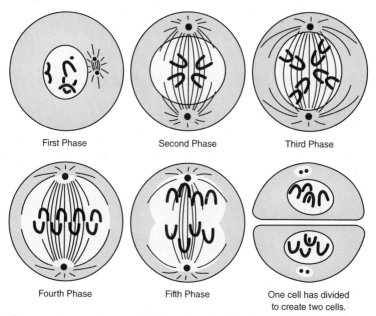

First Phase   Second Phase   Third Phase

Fourth Phase   Fifth Phase   One cell has divided
to create two cells.

Figure 2–2 New cells are created through cell division. Inasmuch, cells are constantly being created and dying. © Milady, a part of Cengage Learning

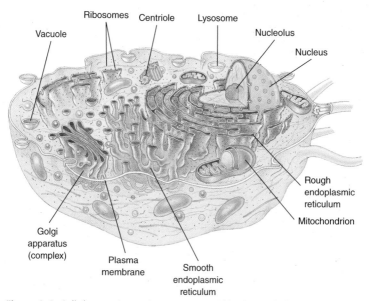

Figure 2–3 Cells have unique microstructures within them which enable the specific cellular function. © Milady, a part of Cengage Learning

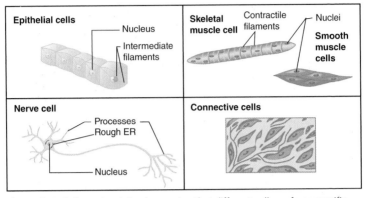

Figure 2–4 Cells are specialized, meaning that different cells perform specific functions within the body. © Milady, a part of Cengage Learning

is developed for a specific reason and plays a role that is necessary to the body; this is called **cell differentiation**. The next level on the ladder of human organization is the organ. Each organ, just like the cells before them, plays a specific role to make the human body function. For example, the circulatory system includes not only the heart but the blood vessels—both arteries and veins—to carry blood throughout the body. The circulatory system could also be called an *organ system*. Other organ systems include the digestive system and the integumentary, or skin, system.

The Cell

The cell is quite complex, but we can consider it to be made up of *three main parts*: the nucleus, the cytoplasm, and the cell membrane. We have learned about the main parts of skin cells, but this structure is true for other cells in the body as well. The nucleus contains the cell's **nucleic acid**, called **DNA** and **RNA**. The nucleus decides what the cell needs and uses the DNA to give instructions for the cellular material to reproduce. As you may know, DNA holds the genetic code for each individual. DNA does not hang loosely within the cell; rather, it is tightly bound by proteins. These proteins are called chromosomes.

The cytoplasm contains many organelles and proteins within the membrane of the cell. Three of the important organelles include mitochondria, golgi apparatus, and lysosomes. These are only three of the important organelles, but you should know that there is a complex organizational process within the cell that allows for cell division. This complex process moves proteins within the cell and creates energy for the cell. The Golgi apparatus is responsible for moving proteins around the cell. Lysosomes clean up the cell and remove the waste. The mitochondrion is the energy center for the cell; it converts carbohydrates from food into energy.

The cell membrane is a structure that protects the cell itself. The membrane can selectively admit or deny admission to the cell, thus protecting the internal environment. The membrane is made of **phospholipids**, which have a complex makeup of carbohydrates and lipids. The cell membrane creates a stable environment for the cell and protects the cell from harm. There are proteins embedded in the cell membrane that send and receive signals to communicate with other cells. The cell also exchanges materials with other cells through the cell membrane using a process called *transport*. The transport process can be either passive transport, such as osmosis, diffusion, and facilitated diffusion; or active transport, which is movement that requires energy.

Human Tissues

Specific cells make up the different human tissues. These tissues work to perform a specific function within the body. As mentioned, there are four types of human tissues: epithelial, connective, muscular, and neural.

Epithelial tissue is found in a continuous sheet of cells with one or more layers. As an aesthetician, you should be familiar with epithelial tissue, as it is also called the skin or simply the **epithelium**. However, epithelial tissues are also found in the linings of the body cavities and major organs. There are several different types of epithelium. The specific types of epithelium include *simple epithelium, squamous epithelial tissue, cuboidal epithelium, columnar epithelial tissue.* Inside the body, the epithelial tissue is also referred to as *endothelium* (Figure 2–5).

Connective tissue is the second in the four types of tissues in the human body. **Connective tissue** is characterized by huge amounts of extracellular matter and intercellular substances and fibers. These fibers should be familiar to the aesthetician and include ground substance and fiber in the form of reticula, collagen, and elastin. The specific combinations of intercellular and extracellular matter result in the different types of connective tissues. The connective tissues help hold the body together and give it support. Connective tissues store minerals and fats as well as allow for motion. There are three types of connective tissues: loose connective tissue, dense connective tissue, and cartilage. Examples of connective tissue include tendons and ligaments.

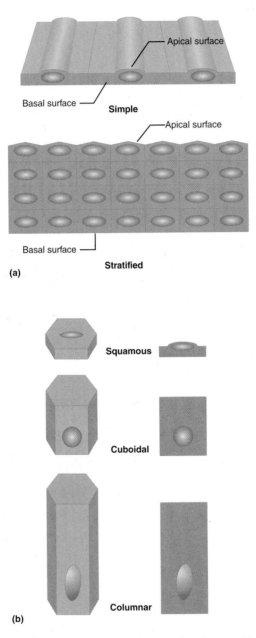

(a)

(b)

Figure 2–5 The cells which make up the skin are referred to as epithelial cells.
© Milady, a part of Cengage Learning

Muscular tissue is divided into three different categories: *skeletal, cardiac,* and *smooth muscle* (Figure 2–6). The **skeletal muscles** are voluntary and typically perpendicular and found attached to bones. The **cardiac muscles** are involuntary and are found in the heart. The **smooth muscle** is involuntary and found throughout the blood vessels and gastrointestinal tract. The purpose of muscle is to promote force or motion within the body. The motion can be thought of in two distinctly different forms: voluntary and involuntary. In the case of **voluntary** muscle movements, these are muscle movements used to move the body forward, such as the movement of the quadriceps of the thigh or the finer movements of the eye. **Involuntary** muscle movement occurs within specific organs, such as the heart or the muscles in the digestive system that push food through the intestines.

Neural cells are found as two cell types within the nervous system. They are the central nervous system, or CNS, and the peripheral nervous system, or PNS. The motor neuron or CNS carries impulses to the muscles and glands, while sensory neurons receive information from the environment.

The Systems and their Organs

Organs are structures that are made of several different types of cells. They each have a specific function and a specific shape. Examples of organs include the heart, the pancreas, the liver, and the lungs. There are 11 different systems within the body, each requiring organs to function (see Figure 2–1).

Skeletal System

This is the system that holds the body erect and supports the internal organs. For example, the brain is protected by the skull. The bones also act as a storehouse for minerals and create new blood cells. This system is divided into two sections: the axial skeleton and the appendicular skeleton. The bones of the **axial skeleton** are those that form the longitudinal axis of the body. Specifically, these are the bones of the skull, the vertebrae, and the thorax. The **appendicular** bones are the bones of the limbs. The skeletal system also includes the joints as well as the cartilages and ligaments that bind the joints together. The joints, of course, allow the body to bend and movement to occur. In addition to providing shape to the body, the skeletal system is also responsible for the support of the body, the protection of the in-ner organs, the movement of the body, the storage of fat and minerals—especially calcium and phosphorus—and, finally, the bones are responsible for the formation of blood. There

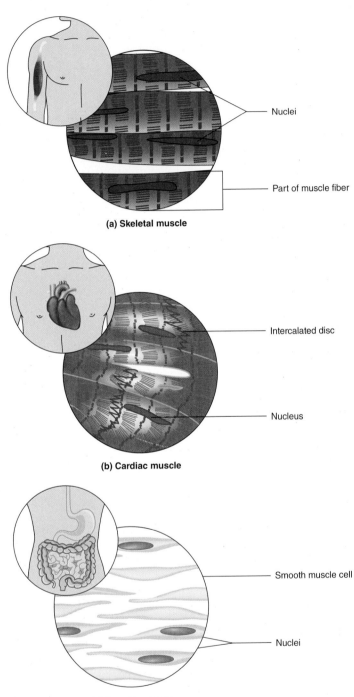

(a) Skeletal muscle

Nuclei

Part of muscle fiber

(b) Cardiac muscle

Intercalated disc

Nucleus

(c) Smooth muscle

Smooth muscle cell

Nuclei

Figure 2–6 Muscle cells make up the many involuntary and voluntary muscles throughout the body. © Milady, a part of Cengage Learning

are four classifications for the bones: long bones, short bones, flat bones, and irregular bones (Figure 2–7). The long bones are those that are longer than they are wide. They are also considered compact. When we think of long bones, we generally consider the bones of the extremities. Short bones are commonly shaped like a cube and are made of a more spongy material than long bones. Examples of short bones include the bones of the wrist and those of the ankle. Flat bones are typically thin, flat, and curved. They contain both spongy and compact material. Examples of flat bones would include the skull, the ribs, and the sternum. The last category of bone type is the irregularly shaped bone. These bones do not fit into other categories and include the hip or pelvis and the vertebrae.

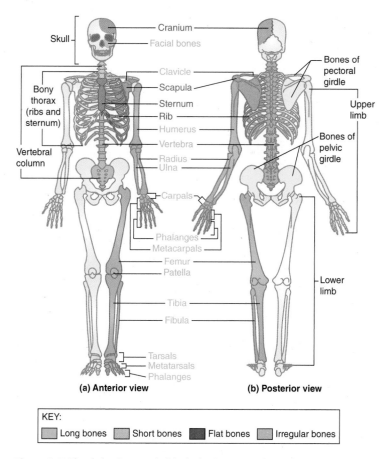

(a) Anterior view   (b) Posterior view

KEY:
■ Long bones   ■ Short bones   ■ Flat bones   ■ Irregular bones

Figure 2–7 The skeletal system holds the body erect and supports the internal organs. © Milady, a part of Cengage Learning

Muscular System

As mentioned earlier, there are three types of muscles found in the human body; they are skeletal, smooth, and cardiac muscle (Figure 2–8). Some of the muscles are defined as voluntary, while others are involuntary muscles. The muscles have four important roles within the body: movement, posture, stabilization of the joints, and generating heat.

Skeletal	Cardiac	Smooth
Attached to bones or, for some facial muscles, to skin	Walls of the heart	Mostly in walls of hollow visceral organs (other than the heart)
Single, very long, cylindrical, multinucleate cells with very obvious striations	Branching chains of cells, uninucleate, striations, intercalated discs	Single, fusiform, uninucleate, no striations

Figure 2–8 Skeletal muscles are striated and voluntary, whereas smooth and cardiac muscles are non-striated and involuntary. © Milady, a part of Cengage Learning

The skeletal muscles which move the body forward by contraction or extension are called voluntary muscles (Figure 2–9). This movement is unique to the skeletal muscles, not appearing in any other system in the body. The large skeletal muscles allow us to move about, as in throwing a ball or running. These muscles have striations which look like lines and are elongated with smooth cells. For this reason, they are defined as **striated** muscle fibers.

The next type of muscle is smooth muscle. This muscle type has no striations and is involuntary; it is the opposite of the skeletal muscle. As it is an involuntary muscle, we have no control of the way it will or will not function. Smooth muscles are found in hollow organs such as the stomach or the bladder.

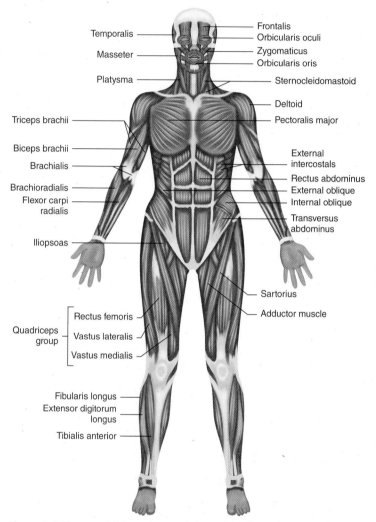

Figure 2–9 The superficial muscles are the ones that allow voluntary or dynamic movement of the body. © Milady, a part of Cengage Learning

This muscle propels substances through a passageway, such as the intestines, to an end point.

The final type of muscle is the cardiac muscle. Since it is cardiac, it is found in only one place in the body and that is the heart. The heart propels blood into the vessels to flow to the organs and systems within the body. Interestingly, while the cardiac muscle is involuntary, it is also striated like skeletal muscle.

Nervous System

The nervous system is the command station for the body. It includes the brain and spinal cord, which are the CNS. The PNS is the nervous system found outside the spinal cord and brain. The CNS is divided into two nerve types: the sensory nerves and the motor nerves (Figure 2–10). The sensory nerves keep the brain informed about what is going on inside and outside the body. The motor nerves cause action from the muscles and glands. The motor nerve has two further subdivisions: the somatic nervous system that allows us to control movement, and the **autonomic nervous system**, which is involuntary (Figure 2–11). Furthermore, there are 12 pairs of **cranial nerves** that serve the head and neck region. The spinal nerves and nerve plexuses number 31; these emanate from the spinal cord. These nerves branch out and serve the body.

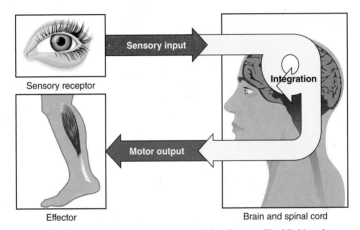

Sensory receptor

Sensory input

Integration

Motor output

Effector

Brain and spinal cord

Figure 2–10 The autonomic nervous system is involuntary, like blinking, but the somatic nervous system is voluntary, like turning your head. Both use nerves that interact with your brain and other physiologic structures. © Milady, a part of Cengage Learning

The nervous system alerts us to problems in our environment. The nervous system is based on immediacy—in a flash it can tell you about external changes such as light or temperature, while the internal nervous system can alert us to a lack of internal oxygen or an increase in carbon dioxide. These alerts come to us via a signal called a *nerve impulse*, which travels along the

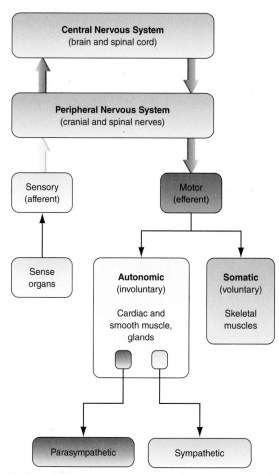

Figure 2–11 The central nervous system plays a vital role in every system in the body.
© Milady, a part of Cengage Learning

nerve (Figure 2–12). The nervous system (brain or spinal cord) assesses the information and then sends a message back through the nervous system for action, such as moving your hand away from a hot flame.

Endocrine System

Like the nervous system, the endocrine system also controls the body's activities. But unlike the nervous system, the **endocrine system** acts slowly with the hormones that are secreted,

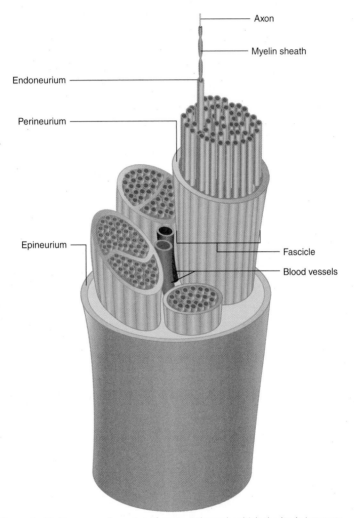

Axon

Myelin sheath

Endoneurium

Perineurium

Epineurium

Fascicle

Blood vessels

Figure 2–12 Nerves are the point of contact through which the body interacts with the outside world. © Milady, a part of Cengage Learning

leisurely making their way through the bloodstream to their destination. The **hormones**, or chemical substances secreted by the endocrine glands, regulate metabolic activity of other cells in the body. The glands we will discuss include the pituitary, thyroid, parathyroid, adrenals, thymus, pancreas, pineal, ovaries in the female, and testes in the male (Figure 2–13). These glands do not connect to one another as in other systems. Rather, they "talk" to other cells in the body via the hormones

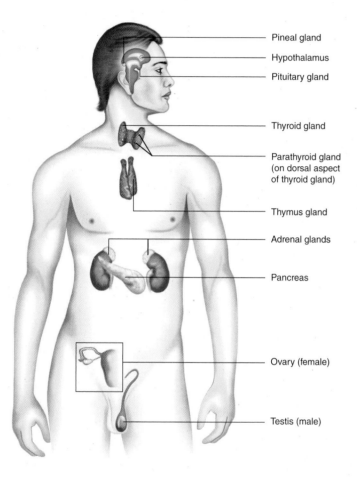

Figure 2–13 Hormones, which regulate many functions within the body, are produced by the endocrine glands. © Milady, a part of Cengage Learning

they release. Hormones are secreted to change the behavior of cells by altering the cellular activity by either increasing or decreasing the rate of the metabolic process. The exact changes depend on the hormone that is secreted and the cell it is connecting to.

Did you know?

The word **hormone** comes from the Greek meaning to arouse.

Though many hormones are produced from the glands noted above, they basically all fall into three categories: amino acid-based molecules, steroids, or prostaglandins. Steroid hormones are made from cholesterol and include the sex hormones, and those hormones made from the adrenal cortex. All the others are nonsteroidal amino acids or prostaglandins.

The **pituitary gland** is about the size of a grape and is found on the interior surface of the hypothalamus of the brain. There are six hormones secreted by the pituitary gland (Figure 2–14). Two of the six hormones secreted by the pituitary gland, the human growth hormone and prolactin, affect nonendocrine cells. The other four hormones affect other endocrine glands, causing them to secrete specific hormones.

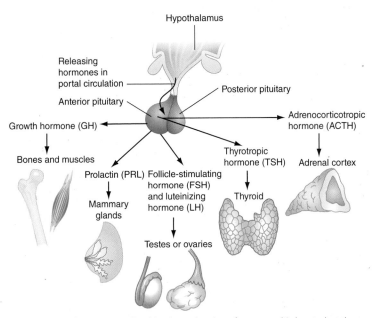

Figure 2–14 The pituitary gland is about the size of a pea and is located at the base of the brain. © Milady, a part of Cengage Learning

The **thyroid** gland is located at the base of the throat (Figure 2–15). It is a large gland compared to some of the other endocrine glands and has two lobes that join together by a central area referred to as the *isthmus*. The thyroid gland makes two hormones, the thyroid hormone and calcitonin.

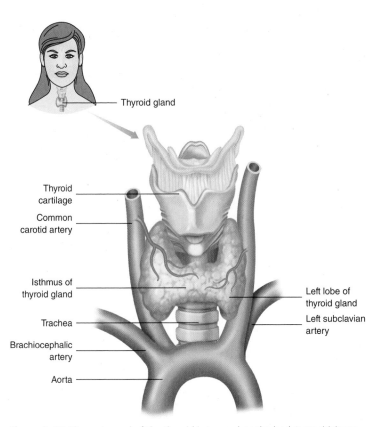

Thyroid gland

Thyroid cartilage

Common carotid artery

Isthmus of thyroid gland

Trachea

Brachiocephalic artery

Aorta

Left lobe of thyroid gland

Left subclavian artery

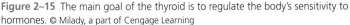

Figure 2–15 The main goal of the thyroid is to regulate the body's sensitivity to hormones. © Milady, a part of Cengage Learning

The *parathyroid* glands are tiny glands found on the posterior side of the thyroid gland. Two glands are typically found on each side of the thyroid, but greater numbers up to eight have been reported. The parathyroid glands secrete parathyroid hormone, also called *parathormone*, which regulates blood calcium levels.

The **adrenal glands** sit on top of the kidneys. The adrenal gland has two distinct areas and functions as two organs. The **adrenal cortex** is the outer covering of the adrenal medulla. The two distinct organs are separated by three separate layers of cells, and each secretes its own hormones. The adrenal cortex secretes three steroids; together they are called the **corticosteroids**. Individually, they are: *mineralocorticoids*, *glucocorticoids*, and *sex hormones*. The adrenal medulla is built of nervous tissue. When it is stimulated by the sympathetic nervous system, it releases two hormones, *adrenaline* and *noradrenaline*. Together, these hormones are known as *catecholamines*. These hormones are the "fight or flight" hormones that are released into the bloodstream when one feels threatened or is being threatened. These hormones increase the blood pressure, the heart rate, and the blood glucose levels and dilate small passageways of the lungs. The catecholamines help the body to prepare or cope with stress.

The **pancreas** is located close to the stomach. The endocrine body within the pancreas is called the *pancreatic islets*. While the pancreas also assists in digestion, it is only the pancreatic islets that we are discussing here. These islets work like an organ within an organ by manufacturing the hormones insulin and glucagons. **Insulin** is the only hormone that can decrease blood glucose levels. Insulin allows the glucose to be accessed by the cell for energy. When the pancreatic islets do not function properly, the client will develop a disease called diabetes mellitus.

Did you know?

When insulin is not available to penetrate the cell and provide energy, the blood glucose level rises to dangerous levels. As it rises, the glucose begins to spill into the urine. As the glucose washes from the body, it is followed by water leading to dehydration. As the glucose spills through the urine, you can smell the sweetness on the breath of the client.

The words **diabetes mellitus** literally mean "something sweet," as the glucose is passing through or siphoned through the kidneys.

Diabetes mellitus comes from the Greek words meaning **something sweet**.

diabetes = siphon

mellitus = honey

Glucagon is a competitor of insulin. It also helps to regulate blood sugar levels, but in the opposite way that insulin does. It increases blood sugar levels. The target of glucagons is the liver, which stores glycogen, which when released into the blood is glucose.

The **pineal gland** is located in the third ventricle of the brain and is somewhat mysterious. While many chemical substances have been identified with the pineal gland, the only hormone known to be excreted by the pineal gland is melatonin. **Melatonin** is believed to be the trigger for sleep.

The **thymus** gland is located in the chest behind the sternum. The hormone produced by the thymus gland is called **thymosin**. During childhood and young adulthood, the thymus acts to harbor and protect a certain white blood cell called a T-lymphocyte or T-cell. These cells are important in the immune process.

The *ovaries* are about the size of almonds and are located in the pelvic cavity. They are specific to the female. The ovaries produce eggs, or *ova*, to be fertilized by the male *sperm* to create offspring. The ovaries produce two steroid hormones: estrogen and progesterone. During puberty, the anterior pituitary hormones send a message to the ovaries to begin to produce the hormones; until that time they are dormant, waiting for the message. **Estrogen** stimulates the female characteristics to form, along with the beginning of the menstrual cycle. **Progesterone** also acts to precipitate the menstrual cycle.

The *testes* are male glands which are suspended in a sac called the scrotum. The testes are not housed in the pelvic cavity like the ovaries. The testes produce the sperm which fertilizes the ova, as previously mentioned. But the testes also create the sex hormones called androgens. Of the androgens produced, *testosterone* is the most important. The **androgens** cause the creation of the primary and secondary male sex characteristics.

Cardiovascular System

When we think of the cardiovascular system, we consider mainly the heart and the blood vessels, both arteries and veins, but blood should also be considered. Blood is the fluid that allows the cardiovascular system to perform its job. The blood is pumped through the heart and lungs, its red blood cells carrying not only oxygen but also nutrients, hormones, and other substances (Figure 2–16). White blood cells, on the other hand, carry bacteria, toxins, and tumor cells for eventual destruction.

The heart is about the size and shape of the fist and weighs less than one pound (Figure 2–17). It is positioned to the left of the chest and on either side of the heart are the lungs. The heart has a double sac of membrane around it called the **pericardium**. Inside against the heart is a thin covering called the **epicardium**. The epicardium is actually part of the heart itself. There are two other layers that compose the heart: the *myocardium* and the *endocardium*.

The heart has four chambers that are hollow. Two are atria and two are ventricles. The **atria** receive the blood and the **ventricles** are the pumps of the heart. The right side works as the pulmonary pump, receiving low-oxygen blood and sending it to the lungs.

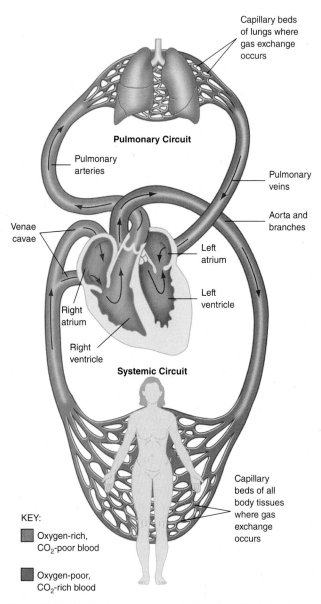

Capillary beds of lungs where gas exchange occurs

Pulmonary Circuit

Pulmonary arteries

Pulmonary veins

Aorta and branches

Venae cavae

Left atrium

Left ventricle

Right atrium

Right ventricle

Systemic Circuit

KEY:

Oxygen-rich, CO_2-poor blood

Oxygen-poor, CO_2-rich blood

Capillary beds of all body tissues where gas exchange occurs

Figure 2–16 The circulatory system carries blood and its vital contents throughout the body. © Milady, a part of Cengage Learning

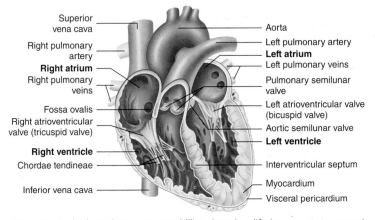

Superior vena cava
Right pulmonary artery
Right atrium
Right pulmonary veins
Fossa ovalis
Right atrioventricular valve (tricuspid valve)
Right ventricle
Chordae tendineae
Inferior vena cava

Aorta
Left pulmonary artery
Left atrium
Left pulmonary veins
Pulmonary semilunar valve
Left atrioventricular valve (bicuspid valve)
Aortic semilunar valve
Left ventricle
Interventricular septum
Myocardium
Visceral pericardium

Figure 2–17 The heart beats over two billion times in a lifetime. © Milady, a part of Cengage Learning

The left side receives the oxygen-rich blood and pumps it to the body. Inside the heart, to prevent the mixing of oxygen-poor and oxygen-rich blood, are valves that are located between the atrial and ventricular chambers on each side. Additional valves are found at the bases of the two large arteries leaving the ventricular chambers. While the heart is loaded with blood all of the time, it does not send blood to the muscle of the heart; this is done through a different circulation pattern called *cardiac circulation.*

The rest of the cardiovascular system is made up of vessels, both arterial and venous (Figure 2–18). These vessels carry the blood to and from the heart, nourishing the tissues with oxygen and taking away carbon dioxide. The blood from the arteries is pushed through the system by the pressure of the heart. The pressure in the veins is low; therefore, veins are assisted by the skeletal muscles and the internal valves to return the blood to the heart (Figure 2–19).

Lymphatic System

The lymphatic system includes the lymphatic vessels, the lymph nodes, the spleen, and the tonsils. The main function of the lymphatic system is to cleanse the blood of toxins and work with other body systems to keep the body's immunity intact.

As blood circulates, the body is exchanging oxygen and carbon dioxide, nutrients and waste. This is done through the fine capillaries and the interstitial fluid (Figure 2–20). Any fluid that is "leaked" in this process is left behind in the fine capillary beds and must be returned to the circulatory system. This is done through the lymphatic system (Figure 2–21). If the

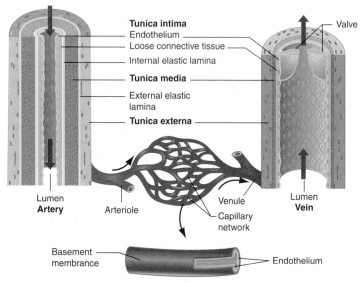

Figure 2–18 The various blood vessels carry the blood from the heart, around the body, and back to the heart. © Milady, a part of Cengage Learning

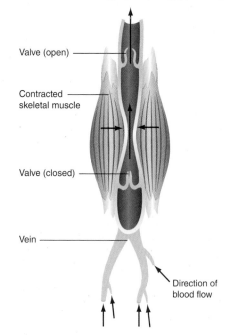

Figure 2–19 Arteries carry oxygenated blood from the heart and veins bring deoxygenated blood back for refueling. © Milady, a part of Cengage Learning

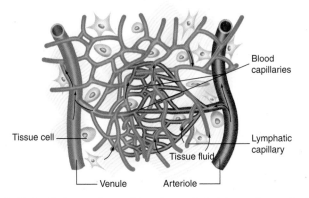

Blood capillaries

Tissue cell

Lymphatic capillary

Tissue fluid

Venule

Arteriole

Figure 2–20 Capillaries are the smallest veins, and arterioles are the smallest arteries. Interstitial fluid is found around the cells of the body and tissues, creating an area called the interstitial space. © Milady, a part of Cengage Learning

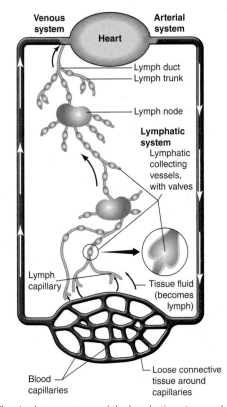

Venous system

Arterial system

Heart

Lymph duct
Lymph trunk

Lymph node

Lymphatic system
Lymphatic collecting vessels, with valves

Lymph capillary

Tissue fluid (becomes lymph)

Blood capillaries

Loose connective tissue around capillaries

Figure 2–21 The circulatory system and the lymphatic system work together to transport toxins away from the body for disposal. © Milady, a part of Cengage Learning

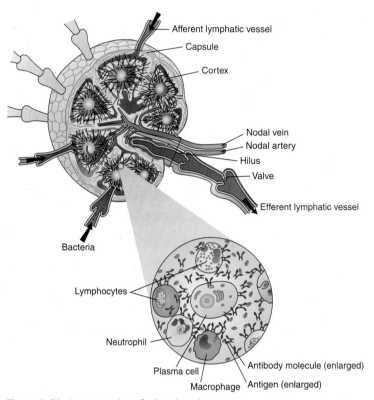

Afferent lymphatic vessel
Capsule
Cortex
Nodal vein
Nodal artery
Hilus
Valve
Efferent lymphatic vessel
Bacteria
Lymphocytes
Neutrophil
Plasma cell
Macrophage
Antibody molecule (enlarged)
Antigen (enlarged)

Figure 2–22 A cross section of a lymph node. © Milady, a part of Cengage Learning

lymphatic system is not working well, **edema** occurs, which can impair the tissues that make the proper exchanges of oxygen and carbon dioxide. The lymphatic vessels are a one-way system, flowing toward the heart. The lymph nodes are more closely associated with the immunity of the body (Figure 2–22). They help to remove foreign debris and bacteria from the body. Examples of this would be bacteria in our bodies when we are sick, which is why our lymph nodes swell. The filtering occurs through **macrophage** cells, which are located in the lymph nodes. The macrophage cells digest the debris and destroy the substance before it can return to the bloodstream. Lymph nodes are only one example of the lymph organs within this system. Other organs that help to purify the blood include the spleen, the tonsils, and the thymus gland, which also produces hormones, as you now know.

As an aesthetician, it is helpful to know that lymphatic drainage can be helpful to the acne client, those with acne-prone skin, and the post-surgical client. As you can see, removing the toxins that are in the body through lymphatic drainage could be an important component of the client's healing process (Figure 2–23).

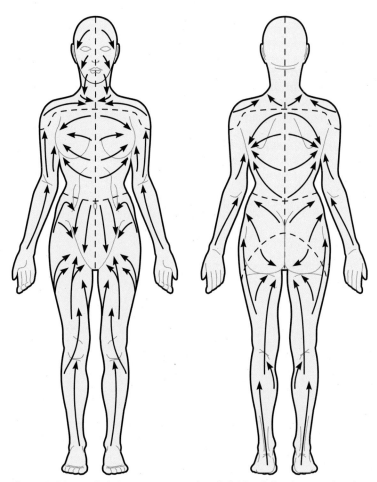

Figure 2–23 Lymph drainage encourages lymph fluid to follow its natural path.
© Milady, a part of Cengage Learning

Respiratory System

The respiratory system supplies the body with oxygen and rids it of carbon dioxide. This system includes the nasal passages, pharynx, larynx, trachea, bronchi, and lungs (Figure 2–24). It is within the lungs that the exchange of oxygen and carbon dioxide is made. The tissues and organs in the body require huge amounts of oxygen to fulfill the cellular functions that make the body work. In fact, the human body cannot do without oxygen even for a few minutes. Further, as the cells use the oxygen supplied to it by the respiratory system they give off carbon dioxide, a waste material for the body that must be gotten rid of. The respiratory system works together with the cardiovascular system, using the blood as the transport fluid, to supply oxygen and take away carbon dioxide (Figure 2–25). The gas exchange itself occurs in the *alveoli*, also called the *terminal sacs*, which are located in the lungs (Figure 2–26). Since the alveoli are the critical and only location for oxygen exchange, the other respiratory system structures are simply the passageways to the alveoli. Nevertheless, the job of the passageways is critical in getting air

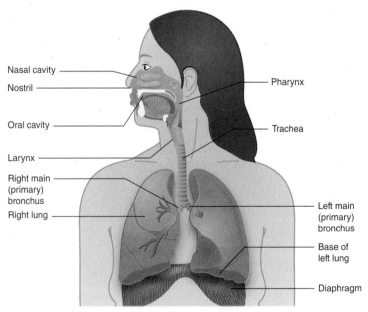

Nasal cavity

Nostril

Oral cavity

Larynx

Right main (primary) bronchus

Right lung

Pharynx

Trachea

Left main (primary) bronchus

Base of left lung

Diaphragm

Figure 2–24 Oxygen is introduced into the body, and carbon dioxide is eliminated by way of expiration. © Milady, a part of Cengage Learning

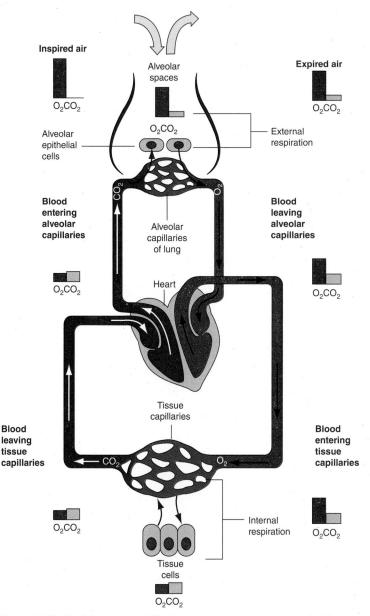

Figure 2–25 All of the organs and body systems require oxygen. It is the blood which supplies them with that oxygen. © Milady, a part of Cengage Learning

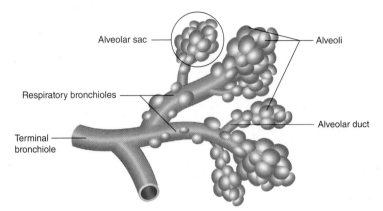

Figure 2–26 Alveloi are little sacs within the lungs wherein the exchange of oxygen and carbon dioxide actually occurs. © Milady, a part of Cengage Learning

to the alveoli. The job of the passageways is to purify, humidify, and warm the incoming air, ensuring that the air is free of dust and bacteria.

Digestive System

The digestive system begins with the *mouth* and ends with the *anus*. The organs of the digestive system include the mouth or oral cavity (including the teeth), the *esophagus, stomach, small intestine*, and *large intestine*, and finally the *rectum*. The main function of the digestive system is to break down the food that is consumed from raw materials (food) into the energy needed to run the body. Specifically, the digestive system ingests the food, digests the food into molecules that the body can use, absorbs the molecules into the bloodstream, and rids the body of the waste through defecation. The digestive system can be broken down into two subsystems. The *alimentary canal* performs the digestive process and contains the accessory digestive organs, which assist with the digestive process (Figure 2–27). The alimentary canal is more commonly known as the *gastrointestinal* or GI tract. It is a long winding tube that is open at both ends (Figure 2–28). The organs associated with the GI tract include the mouth, pharynx, esophagus, stomach, small intestine, and large intestine. The GI tract begins at the mouth and ends at the anus. The accessory organs of digestion include the *salivary glands*, the *teeth*, the pancreas, the *liver*, and the *gallbladder*. The salivary glands empty their contents into the mouth through the *parotid glands*, which are anterior to the ears.

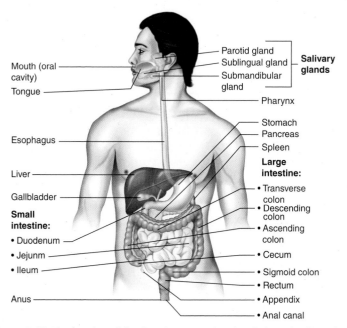

Figure 2–27 The function of the digestive system is to break down food into fuel for energy. © Milady, a part of Cengage Learning

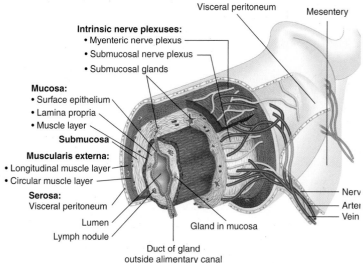

Figure 2–28 The alimentary canal is more commonly known as the gastrointestinal (GI) tract. It is here that digestion actually occurs. © Milady, a part of Cengage Learning

There are also salivary glands in the *submandibular* (under the mandible) and **sublingual** (under the tongue) areas. The salivary glands release an enzyme called *salivary amylase*, which begins the process of digestion. The teeth tear the food apart and mix the food with salivary amylase to assist in the digestion process. The pancreas is involved in maintaining blood glucose levels, as we have already discovered, but the pancreas also has other functions, among them the production of enzymes that break down the food for digestion. The enzymes that are secreted from the pancreas are alkaline in nature. These alkaline enzymes neutralize the stomach's acidic enzymes to further the digestive process. The liver is the largest gland in the body and is intimately involved in the digestive process. Located under the diaphragm and slightly to the right, the liver is one of the body's most important organs. It has many metabolic roles, but in the digestive process, its purpose is to secrete *bile*. The gallbladder is located on the interior surface of the liver. The gallbladder stores bile for later use.

Urinary System

Waste is produced throughout the body. The urinary system is responsible for removing nitrogen-containing wastes from the blood, pushing them through the urinary or excretory system. This system includes the *kidneys, ureters, bladder,* and *urethra* (Figure 2–29). This system is also responsible for the balance of salt and water within the body.

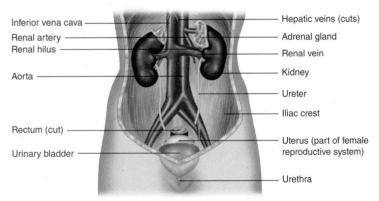

Figure 2–29 The urinary system transports waste and excess minerals out of the body. © Milady, a part of Cengage Learning

The kidneys are responsible for the purity of the body. Their job is to filter water from the blood and process the water, eliminating waste through the urinary system. Interestingly, the lungs and the skin (through perspiration) play a role in the process of excretion. But it is primarily the kidneys that are responsible for the elimination of nitrogen-containing waste, toxins, and some drugs from the body. As the kidneys manage the water waste through the body, they maintain the volume of blood that is circulating. The kidneys also produce an enzyme called *renin*, which helps to maintain blood pressure. The kidneys are the only functioning organs of the urinary system (Figure 2–30). The other organs—the bladder and ureters and urethra—are simply storage areas and passageways for the urine.

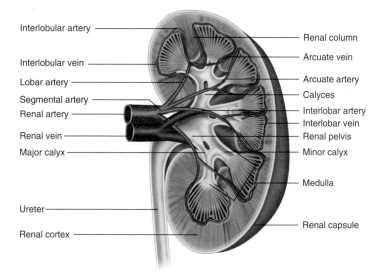

Figure 2–30 The kidneys are the only functioning organs of the urinary system.
© Milady, a part of Cengage Learning

Reproductive System

This is the system that is present only to produce offspring. Sperm are produced by the male gonads called the *testes*. Other male reproductive organs include the scrotum, penis, and accessory glands and duct work (Figure 2–31). This duct work carries the sperm out of the body and into the female to fertilize eggs, thus creating a new human being. The organs of

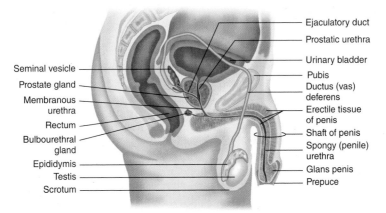

Figure 2–31 The male reproductive organs produce and emit sperms cells, the specialized cells which fertilize the egg. © Milady, a part of Cengage Learning

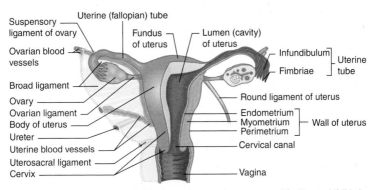

Figure 2–32 The female reproductive organs produce eggs and facilitate childbirth. © Milady, a part of Cengage Learning

reproduction for the female include the duct system that connects the ovaries to the uterus, the uterus itself, and the vagina (Figure 2–32).

Unlike all of the other systems in the body, the reproductive system plays no specific role in sustaining life. In fact, up until puberty, the reproductive system is basically asleep, waiting for the call to action. The hormones produced by the reproductive organs play vital roles in the development of the girl into a woman and the boy into a man. Those hormones, previously discussed, are also important for the development of the organs of reproduction, sexual behavior, and libido.

An Overview of the Skin

The skin and its appendages—nails, hair, nerve endings, sweat and oil glands—collectively encompass the **integumentary system**, sometimes referred to as *integument* (Figure 2–33). Skin is vital to our survival, as it keeps our bodies and its various components intact and, just as importantly, provides our immediate contact with the environment. Our skin senses vital information about the world in which we live; therefore, it ensures our survival. Although seemingly uniform and simple in its presentation and purpose, it is far more complex and variant than meets the eye. Skin varies in thickness and in sensitivity.

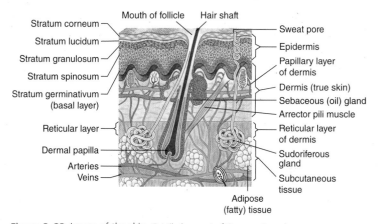

Figure 2–33 Layers of the skin. © Milady, a part of Cengage Learning

Despite its significance in our health, appearance, and well-being, skin may be the most disregarded organ of the body. Damage can range from annoying to life-threatening (going beyond simple aging to include disease). Infections can be bacterial, fungal, parasitic, and viral. Various forms of **dermatitis** produce fluid-filled vesicles on the skin surface. Any slow-healing or encrusted lesions of the skin, as well as lesions that **suppurate** (discharge), should alert us to the strong possibility of pathogens. As aestheticians providing treatments it is important for us to recognize potential skin problems, know the limitations of our treatments, and know when to seek help for our clients.

Although seemingly uniform and simple in its presentation and purpose, skin is far more complex and variant than meets the eye. Skin varies in thickness and in sensitivity. During development in the womb, parts of it develop from brain tissue and become attached to the brain through nerves, which conduct pleasure and pain.[1] These signals are vital to our success as a species. Although not all of the sensations humans feel are pleasurable, they are all purposeful. If we could not sense cold air, we would all freeze to death. If we could not feel a cut, we could bleed to death or die from infection. These sensations are sensed by nerves, which in turn send the information to our brains for processing and translation. Overall, the skin possesses most of the nerve endings that transmit vital information about our environment to the brain. Relatively few are found on our posterior sides; however, in lips, fingers, and genitals, they are abundant.

Because the skin is our outermost organ, it also serves as a unique identifier, which we see and use to associate and differentiate one person from another. Being the psychosocial creatures we are, we have put great emphasis on how others perceive the way we appear. The way we dress, decorate, and posture ourselves conveys gender, age, strength, and most noticeably, attractiveness.

The appearance of the skin has become a synonym for beauty in our society, and we strive to optimize it. New scientific developments promise creams that act longer, stronger, or faster to turn back the clock. Some consumers are extraordinarily sophisticated in finding the newest treatments and the latest products to counteract the aging process. Others are overwhelmed by the options available to them. Either way, we can do things to maintain and even regain beautiful skin (Table 2–1). To do so we must ask ourselves questions: How do we determine what works best? Why does it work? How much change is possible? Even the savviest consumer needs help answering these questions. Most of them will turn to you for advice. It is here that our quest begins.

Did you know?

An active organ, the skin provides protection, conveys sensation, sends signals, regulates temperature, produces vitamin D_3, and helps rid our bodies of unneeded or threatening components.[2] It is elastic—it stretches when we frown or smile or bend, and regains its normality when we relax.[3]

TABLE 2–1 Fun Facts About the Skin[4]

Humans shed millions of dead skin flakes every minute.
In adults, the skin usually covers about 2 m² (about the size of a shower curtain) and weighs about 7 lbs. It also has 300 million skin cells.
The skin is between 1.5 mm and 4 mm thick, about as thick as a few sheets of paper.
The thickest areas of the skin (plantar and palmar regions) contain no hair follicles or sweat glands.
Millions of coiled sweat glands discharge sweat and salts to the surface, where evaporation begins to cool the body in seconds.
Just below the surface, the dermis feeds miles of blood vessels with nutrients.
The brain and skin become connected very early in fetal development. Even in the womb, a baby's hand can feel its way to the mouth.
Touch is the first sense to develop.
The skin's array of nerves is sensitive enough to feel the weight of a mosquito as it lands.

Skin Physiology

As discussed, the skin does much more than just hold in the other organs. Not much thicker than a sheet of paper, skin is quite complex. In general terms, it protects, senses, and aids temperature regulation, excretion, immunologic response, and metabolism.

Protection

Protection is one of the skin's main functions. Skin acts as a barrier against intruders such as water, ultraviolet light, bacteria, and fungi. It also protects vital organs against minor trauma. The skin is a mostly waterproof sheath that guards against too much moisture entering or escaping from the body. It also secretes acids that could otherwise allow bacteria and viruses to penetrate our skin and cause disease or even death.[5] Likewise, the skin acts as armor against foreign matter. The final way the skin protects us is against the damaging effects of solar rays. The pigment melanin is produced as an active response to ultraviolet light, thus preventing cellular damage. This will be discussed in more detail later in this chapter.

Sensation and Communication

Skin is capable of receiving a diverse amount of tactile information from a variety of receptors. *Neural receptors*, some of them quite elaborate, mediate touch, position, pressure, temperature, and pain. The communication goes two ways and occurs instinctively. The skin releases signals such as blushing, **pheromones** (unique chemical signals), and body odor.

The four senses recognized by the skin are (1) touch (pressure being sustained by contact), (2) cold, (3) heat, and (4) pain[6] (Figure 2–34). Nerves that receive and send these sensory signals to the brain show a variety of sensory endings, including expanded tips (Merkel's disks and Ruffini's endings), encapsulated endings (Pacinian corpuscles, **Meissner's corpuscles**, and Krause's end-bulbs), and simple naked nerve endings. Many sensory nerves terminate around hair follicles. Expanded or encapsulated nerve endings can also occur in areas of the body removed from the skin—explaining *deep* pain we can feel, such as a kidney punch.

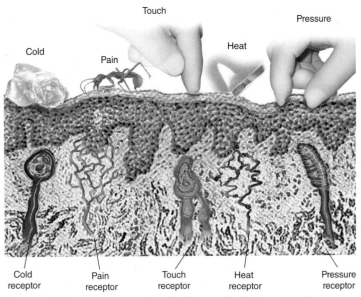

Figure 2–34 Sensory nerve endings. © Milady, a part of Cengage Learning

Thermoregulation

Skin is critical for regulating body temperature.[7] The body's optimal internal (or *core*) temperature is maintained by actions of blood vessels in the lower layer of the skin. Blood vessels will insulate the body's core temperature from both internal and external temperature variations by constricting and relaxing blood flow. When we are exposed to cold, blood vessels in the lower layer of the skin constrict. This allows the blood to bypass that which would cool it as the skin cools to the outside temperature. When it is warm, those blood vessels dilate and heat is radiated outward. Perspiration evaporates off the surface of the skin and cools us. To this effect, body heat is conserved.

Although normal core body temperature is 37° C, or 98.6° F, skin surface is normally cooler, around 33° C, or 91° F.[8] The surface temperature of the skin depends on the temperature of the air that touches it and the amount of time spent in that air. Weather factors such as wind and humidity affect skin temperature, and temperatures at different points of the skin surface can differ dramatically. After exertions on a windy and snowy day, one climber on Denali (Mt. McKinley) reported the temperature of his big toe to be 42° F at the same time that the surface of his chest measured 88° F.[9]

Metabolism

Blood vessels within the lower layer of the skin also provide nutrition for the skin. Blood flow carries vitamins, minerals, and oxygen that are critical to the skin's health and appearance. Oxygen requirements for skin are *greater* than those of connective tissue, and if not enough oxygen is supplied, the health of the skin may suffer. This is why smoking cigarettes may cause problems with healing. Skin health not only affects how we look but also how quickly and smoothly injuries such as cat scratches and paper cuts heal.

Immunologic Response

Skin contains specialized cells to protect it and all of the elements it contains. Mast cells and Langerhans cells defend the skin against microorganisms. *Langerhans cells* detect antigens in the uppermost layer of the skin. **Mast cells** are poised to create an inflammatory response should the skin be injured.[10] This is evidenced by allergic reactions. Mast cells are responsible for histamine and related responses to mosquito bites and bee stings.

Excretion

The skin releases fluid and toxins through the sweat glands. These same glands are important regulators of body temperature, as mentioned previously.[11]

Skin Anatomy

If one of the skin's main functions is to act as a barrier against intruding substances, then how do lotions that we apply absorb into the skin? The main answer is the appendages. **Appendages** are smaller parts of a greater part. For the skin, they include the **pilosebaceous unit** (hair follicle and accompanying sebaceous glands and arrector pili muscle), sweat glands, and nails.[12] Appendages originate in the uppermost layer of the skin (the **epidermis**) but extend in pockets of epidermis into the lower layer, the **dermis**.

External substances such as skin creams, ointments, and salves can enter the skin through the appendages of the hair and sweat glands through the intercellular spaces between the cornified cells, or smaller molecules can pass through cells at the surface of the skin.

Sweat Glands

You can think of sweat glands as simple tubes. They are vital for regulating body temperature. Because of the composition of what they carry to the surface, sweat glands also influence water balance and ionic penetration.

Ordinary **eccrine sweat glands** are located over most of the body, and large **apocrine sweat glands** are concentrated in axillary (underarm), pubic, and perianal areas.[13] The latter develop at puberty.[14] Although sweat from the apocrine glands is initially odorless, it can mix with bacteria on the skin and acquire an odor.

> The skin's appendages are important in healing, especially superficial healing and protection of the skin. When the skin is superficially injured over a limited surface, it can grow back quickly because of **epithelial cells** remaining in deeper hair follicles and sweat glands.

Normal, healthy adults secrete about one pint of sweat per day (more with physical activity).[15] Because of daily loss of water, everyone needs to actively replace water lost inside the body regardless of their activity level. However, the more active you are, the more water needs to be replaced. As much as four cups of water can be lost during hard exercise. To avoid dehydration, water should be consumed regularly throughout the day and more before, during, and after exercise. When a person has become thirsty, he or she is already dehydrated, so it is important to consume fluids regardless of thirst. Symptoms of dehydration include dizziness, disorientation, and clumsiness.[16]

Hair Follicles

Hair is a type of modified skin. It grows everywhere on a person's body except the palmar and plantar regions of hands and feet. *Hair follicles* are densest on the head, neck, and shoulder regions, where there can be as many as 300 to 900/cm^2. Conversely, about 100/cm^2 are found on the torso and limbs.[17] Hair follicles are tubular (Figure 2–35). They extend deep into the skin to develop and nourish the hair. The hair follicle contains epidermal cells, whereas the hair itself is **keratin**. Hair follicles have several distinct anatomic components, including the *bulb*, the *root*, and the *papilla*.

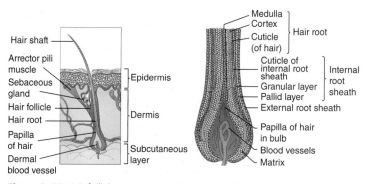

Figure 2–35 Hair follicle structure. © Milady, a part of Cengage Learning

The hair follicle, gland, nerve, and muscle are called the pilosebaceous unit. Hair follicles are associated with **sebaceous glands** (small masses of cells and fat associated with hair follicles) that lubricate the hair; nerve endings that detect motion of the hair shaft and control *piloerection* ("goose bumps"); and smooth muscle, which actually creates the goose bumps.[18]

The sebaceous glands which are most active reside on the face, chest, and back.

All hair goes through an **anagen phase** (growing), a **catagen phase** (transitional), and a **telogen phase** (resting)—the hair grows, resides for a while, and then falls out.[19] This growth cycle varies in different parts of the body. For instance, the entire cycle takes four months for eyelashes and three to four years for hair on the scalp.

As we will see, this process of division, growth, and maturation somewhat resembles that of the skin's top layer. In both cases, cells go through a process of hardening and then **sloughing**, or being shed. However, when cells at the bottom of the hair follicle slough, they create a column of **keratinized** (hardened, "horny") cells. This is the hair that grows up through the shaft and extends through the follicle. Hair growth is a complex process, but understanding this process is key to the success of hair removal with lasers or light. Lasers are known to be effective only on hairs in the growth (anagen) phase.

Nails

Like hair, nails are also a type of modified skin.[20] They are formed from hardened cells in the top layer of skin (Figure 2–36). Nails on the fingers and toes protect their sensitive tips. They provide support for the tips of our digits and assist in picking up objects. Although effective, they are not necessary for living (and neither are details of their histology necessary for us to know).

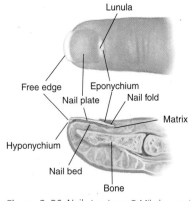

Figure 2–36 Nail structure. © Milady, a part of Cengage Learning

Layers of the Skin

The skin is comprised of two main layers: (1) the epidermis and (2) the dermis. The epidermis, or top layer, is tough and, because of its exposure, constantly being worn down and replaced.[21] It contains no blood vessels or nerves and is vital in preventing loss of moisture from the body. The deeper layer of the skin, the dermis, and the **subcutaneous** (meaning *beneath* the skin) fat beneath it lend strength and elasticity to the skin. Within both layers of skin are sublayers, each with cells that perform specific functions.

Epidermis

The epidermis is the skin that we see (Figure 2–37). It contains tiny pockets that house sweat glands and pilosebaceous glands.[22] Compared to the dermis, it is often very thin, approximately 0.12 mm, but its thickness also varies dramatically over the body.[23] It is thickest on the palms of the hands and soles of the feet and thinnest on the eyelids.

The epidermis is **avascular** (without blood vessels), impermeable to water, physically tough, and dry at the surface to impede the growth of microorganisms. It is continually replacing itself. When the epidermis is injured or diseased, its replacement speeds up in response; this is important to us as aestheticians. In short, it is our self-replicating defense against everything outside of us.

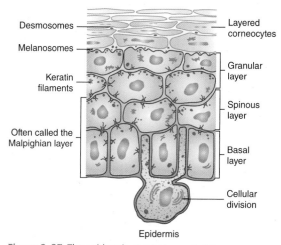

Desmosomes — Layered corneocytes
Melanosomes
Keratin filaments — Granular layer
— Spinous layer
Often called the Malpighian layer — Basal layer
— Cellular division

Epidermis

Figure 2–37 The epidermis. © Milady, a part of Cengage Learning

As the outermost layer of the skin, the epidermis shields us from the environment, potential injury, bacteria, pollution, and most everything else that wants to penetrate it. The dermis is the support, providing the epidermis with strength and stability.

Unlike other cellular components of the body, such as nerves, epidermal cells are born, die, and are replaced by new ones. If all of the cells of the body behaved like those of the epidermis, there would be no spinal cord paralysis or diabetes, because cellular renewal would solve those injuries and diseases.

Within the epidermis are five less distinct *sublayers*. These sublayers are not composed of different cell *types*; instead, they reflect *stages* of hardening, maturation, and eventual death in the migration of their major cell type, the keratinocyte.[24]

The different stages are called the **cell differentiation** (Figure 2–38). The sublayers of the epidermis include, from the top, the stratum corneum, the stratum lucidum, the stratum granulosum, the stratum spinosum, and the stratum basale.

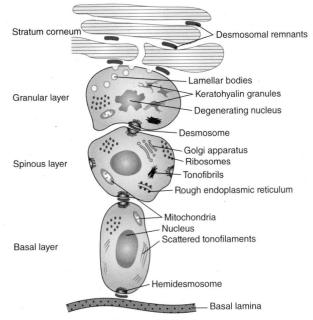

Figure 2–38 This is cell differentiation. © Milady, a part of Cengage Learning

Stratum Corneum

The **stratum corneum** is the *top* or superficial layer of the epidermis. It varies in thickness: thin on the upper arm; thick on the soles, palms, and areas of chronic friction. Its thickness can be affected by simple dry skin and by disease processes such as psoriasis.

Each month, the cells of the **stratum basale**, or the basal layer (bottom layer of the epidermis), make their way through the layers of the epidermis into the stratum corneum. The cells begin as healthy plump cells with fully functioning nuclei. However, as they near the summit they shrivel and flatten out.[25] The cells complete their gradual transition to death and are soon sloughed off, but this is what makes them protective.

Unbeknownst to us, our bodies gently and constantly lose water via evaporation through a process called **transepidermal water loss (TEWL)**.[26] When too much water evaporates, not only our skin but also our bodies suffer ill effects. Preventing excessive water loss is important both to the skin and to the body as a whole.

Although it is drier than lower skin layers, the **stratum corneum** contains a compound, **natural moisturizing factor** (NMF), that helps to keep the skin soft and moisturized even in dry climates.[27] NMF is composed of amino acids and **filaggrin,** water-soluble chemicals capable of absorbing large quantities of water. The presence of NMF in the stratum corneum is critical for soft and flexible skin. Although NMF is contained only in the uppermost layer of the skin, its existence is made possible by ingredients provided by deeper structures.[28]

NMF gives the cells of the stratum corneum their ability to bind with water. NMF is found only in the stratum corneum and is solely responsible for the regulation of water in the very superficial layers of the stratum corneum. Not surprisingly, its presence is diminished by age and excessive exposure to soap. This is key to understanding the phenomenon of dry skin.

In the stratum corneum, filaggrin assists keratinocytes in creating the NMF. Later, it combines with other cells found within the granular layer to create strength and stability for the epidermis.

It is worth noting that NMF and TEWL have nothing to do with water loss associated with sweating. It is a common misconception that drinking water will improve hydration levels of the skin. This is simply not true. Drinking water improves water level inside the body, but is used up there. The best way to rehydrate the skin is by applying a topical moisturizer.

Stratum Lucidum

This thin, clear band (*lucidum* means *clear* or *bright*) of closely packed cells is most prominent in areas of thick skin and may be absent in other areas.[29]

Stratum Granulosum

Like the other sublayers of the epidermis, this layer signals transition of the cells within it.[30] It is in this layer that the keratin loses nuclei and organelles, becoming flat before moving farther up into the stratum corneum. It is called the *stratum granulosum* because of the granules that now appear in the cells. In effect, these granules write the death warrant of the cell, because as the granules grow in size, the nucleus—the power generator of the cell—disintegrates and dies.[31]

Stratum Spinosum

Stratum spinosum means spiny layer. Cells in this sublayer are intertwined with tiny structures called **desmosomes**. Under the microscope, desmosomes resemble hair combed with an eggbeater, which is why this part is often called the *prickly cell* layer. The hairlike desmosomes permit materials to move around them in the intercellular space. **Lamellar granules** are also found here. These granules control lipids that migrate to the stratum corneum and become another component of NMF.

In this, the first leg of the journey, keratinocytes depart the basal layer and show the first signs of keratinization. Here also we find lamellar granules, organelles that deliver fats to the stratum corneum. These granules contain the lipids and other components such as cholesterol, fatty acids, ceramides, and enzymes necessary to produce NMF. Once these granules reach the stratum corneum they release their contents and cause the NMF to occur.

Stratum Basale

The "basement" of the epidermis is appropriately called the *basal layer*. It anchors the epidermis to the dermis. This layer contains **germinal cells**—cells of regeneration—for all sublayers of the epidermis. It is here that few different basal cell types are housed, including stem cells, amplifying cells, and postmitotic cells. Basal cells remain in the basal layer, creating a solid skin foundation, and keratinocytes begin their upward migration to the stratum corneum.

Specialized Epidermal Cells

Four specialized cells exist within the epidermis: (1) keratinocytes, (2) melanocytes, (3) Langerhans cells, and (4) Merkel cells (Table 2–2).

TABLE 2–2 Specialized Epidermal Cells

Cell Type	Location	Function
Keratinocytes	Generated in the strata basale; half begin to migrate upward, eventually to be sloughed off	Basic skin cells that collectively make up skin; undergo desquamation
Melanocytes	Between epidermis and dermis	Secrete pigments that give skin, hair, and eyes their color
Langerhans cells	Strata spinosum and strata basale	Patrol epidermis for foreign invaders; ingest them for removal by the lymphatic system
Merkel cells	By nerve endings throughout epidermis	Exact function unclear; likely involved in sensation

Keratinocytes

Keratinocytes are cells that are usually close to nerve endings and may be involved in sensory perception. The majority of cells in the epidermis are keratinocytes. These cells are generated in the basal sublayer but destined, half the time, to depart. Fifty percent of the keratinocytes produced remain in the basal sublayer of the epidermis (and are then, as you saw previously, identified as basal cells). The others, retaining their keratinocyte identity and a certain apparent ambition, begin moving up, passing through the remaining sublayers to the surface, then becoming hard and cornified, and finally being sloughed off.[32]

During differentiation, keratinocytes go through critical changes. The shape flattens, then organelles are "lost" and fibrous proteins are shaped, and finally, as the cell becomes dehydrated, the cell membrane thickens.

The process of moving from the basal layer to the stratum corneum and then sloughing off is called **desquamation**. It takes approximately 28 to 35 days in younger people and up to 45 days as we age. When it takes longer, it shows. Delays in the migration process and extrinsic factors such as smoking, solar damage, and pollution cause the skin to turn sallow and gray.

Melanocytes

Located in or near the basal layer, **melanocytes** (Figure 2–39) occupy the junction between the epidermis and the dermis. They secrete the pigment **melanin** that lends color to skin, eyes, and hair. Melanin protects the skin from ultraviolet light and is produced in response to it. Melanin is also produced in response to genetic and hormonal cues, such as a pregnancy. Skin color is not determined by melanocyte concentration or quantity, but rather by the degree of melanocyte activity. Men and women of all races have roughly equal amounts of melanocytes.

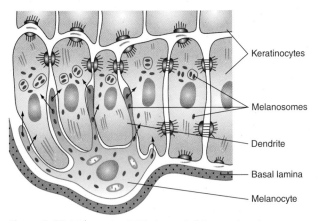

Figure 2–39 Melanocyte. © Milady, a part of Cengage Learning

The faster the keratinocyte moves to the stratum corneum, the more youthful skin appears. Through the use of microdermabrasion, our objective is to increase the migration rate of keratinocytes to the stratum corneum without injuring the skin.

After melanocytes have produced melanin, they transfer it to keratinocytes via small appendages that act like eyedroppers. Regardless of whether they carry cargo, keratinocytes continue their migration toward the surface.[33] In this cellular relationship, melanocytes are the melanin-*making* cell and keratinocytes are the melanin-*receiving* cell; although melanocytes produce melanin, in the end keratinocytes contain it. The proportion of melanocytes to keratinocytes varies from 1:4 to 1:10, depending on age, with melanocyte proportion decreasing with age. Therefore, our ability to protect our skin with melanin decreases as we get older.

> Although melanocytes partially protect the skin from ultraviolet radiation, do not be fooled into thinking that those who tan easily or have darker skin types are protected from skin cancers.

Both injury and inflammation can cause increases in melanin production. Such an injury is known as **post-inflammatory hyperpigmentation** and is a recognized complication of both microdermabrasion and peeling.

Langerhans Cells

Found in the lower layers of the epidermis, Langerhans cells engage in surveillance against would-be intruders.[34] Although smaller in breadth than keratinocytes, they stretch fingerlike processes between keratinocytes to the surface, where they scan like periscopes. Upon encountering "bad bacteria," they *acquire* them and transport the offenders to T-lymphocytes in the regional lymph nodes for disposal.

Merkel Cells

Merkel cells are associated with the nerve endings found in the epidermis. Their specific function remains unclear, but because they are numerous about the lips, hard palate, palms, finger- and footpads, and proximal nail folds, they are likely involved in sensation.[35,36]

Dermis

In our continued exploration of the skin, we encounter the second, deeper layer—the dermis (Figure 2–40). The dermis provides the vital function of attaching skin to body.

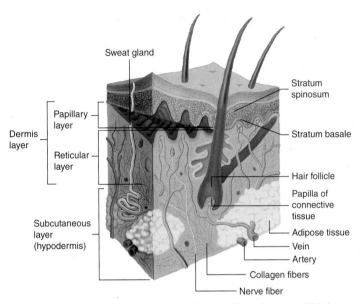

Figure 2–40 The dermis has two layers: (1) the papillary dermis, and (2) the reticular dermis. Beneath the reticular dermis lies the hypodermis, or subcutaneous fat. © Milady, a part of Cengage Learning

The dermis is crisscrossed with three types of fibers that lend strength and elasticity. These fibers—reticulin, collagen, and elastin—form a network that creates stability for the skin. Type I collagen runs throughout the dermis and is responsible for its tensile strength and for providing skin with its youthful appearance of tightness, firmness, and fullness.[37] The combined strength of these tissues anchors the epidermis above to the subcutaneous tissue below.

Epidermal appendages such as sweat glands and hair follicles are embedded in the dermis, which also serves as the end point for blood vessels and nerves.[38]

On its superficial side, the dermis holds the epidermis at the **dermal-epidermal junction (DEJ)**. On its distal side, it attaches to subcutaneous tissue.

The dermis, which varies in thickness but is typically about 2 ml thick, is further subdivided into the papillary and reticular layers.[39] This subdivision is based on differences in collagen texture.[40]

Papillary Dermis

The **papillary dermis**, the most superficial layer of the dermis, is the first skin layer to contain capillary blood vessels, small nerves, and lymphatic vessels.

Because the papillary dermis contains blood vessels and blood vessels provide temperature changes when they constrict or dilate, it is the papillary dermis that is specifically responsible for thermoregulation of the body. When you are performing microdermabrasion and encounter *pinpoint bleeding*, you have arrived at the papillary dermis. Does that not increase your respect for the thickness of the epidermis?

> Collagen in the papillary dermis is finely textured.[41] It contains projections called **papillae**, which fit the dermis to the epidermis.[42] We are accustomed to using these uniquely individual ridged patterns in foot- and fingerprinting.[43]

In addition to its *holding* properties, the papillary dermis has another very important function in regulating the appearance of skin surface—it houses **glycosaminoglycans (GAGs)**. GAGs are a variety of *chains* made of polysaccharide, a type of complex carbohydrate. Attracted almost fanatically to water, GAGs are thought capable of binding up to 1000 times their weight in water.[44] Think for a moment about the padding this provides. This moisture-attracting property makes them one of the most important components in our study of the skin. Unfortunately, many histology studies of the skin show a decrease in the number of GAGs with age.[45]

Reticular Dermis

The **reticular dermis** is located beneath the papillary dermis and rests on the thick pad of fat known as subcutaneous tissue. Here lies the real anchor of the skin.

> Collagen in this layer (**reticular** means like a network) is larger and more coarsely textured.[46] In the example of a cow's skin after tanning, it is the cow's dermis that makes the leather.[47]

Within the reticular dermis are structures called **rete pegs**. These "pegs" extend up into the epidermis (and similar structures extend from above down into the dermis) to hold the dermis to the epidermis. These structures are responsible for holding the epidermis and dermis together to create the skin. Capillary networks run through rete pegs like tiny elevators, bringing nutrients to the epidermis. It is widened vessels in the rete pegs that cause broken capillaries. People with transparent or very light skin may flush or blush, causing a dilation of the capillaries in the rete pegs.

> The reticular dermis houses the appendages of the skin, nerves, and blood vessels. It is loaded with collagen, blood vessels, and nerve endings.

Specialized Dermal Cells

Many **specialized dermal** cells exist. Their functions range from directing the production of collagen and ground substance to providing nutrients and removing waste from the skin (Table 2–3).

TABLE 2–3 Specialized Dermal Cells

Cell Type	Location	Function
Fibroblasts	Reticular dermis, papillary dermis	Direct the production of collagen, reticulin, and ground substance
Mast cells	Papillary dermis	Protect skin against invasion and infection
Ground substance	Reticular dermis, papillary dermis	Provide nutrients and remove waste

Fibroblast Cells

Fibroblasts are the *command* cells for the dermis. They direct the production of collagen, elastin, and reticulin and the ground substance for the dermis. In response to injury, fibroblasts proliferate to manufacture new collagen, from which scarring occurs.[48]

Mast Cells

Along with lymphocytes and macrophages, the mast cells reside in connective tissue of the dermis, usually in the neighborhood of blood vessels. These cells protect against injury and invasion. Release of **histamine** by mast cells produces the inflammation that ousts intruders and begins wound healing.[49] In allergic reactions manifested in the skin, such as hives, large numbers of mast cells exist. We would see this in a condition such as **urticaria pigmentosa**.

Ground Substance

Through diffusion, **ground substance** provides nutrients to and removes wastes from other tissue components.[50] It is integral to the healing process. As a wound heals, the available ground substance creates a moister wound that will heal more quickly. It is constantly undergoing synthesis and degradation. The ground substance of the dermis consists largely of GAGs. Age probably brings a decrease in ground substance.

Hypodermis or Subcutaneous Tissue

Under the reticular dermis lies the **hypodermis**, or subcutaneous fat. It is made up of clumps of fat-filled cells called **adipose** cells. It is the "cushion layer" of the skin and helps protect internal organs from blows; it also acts as an insulator, conserving body heat.[51]

The attachment of subcutaneous tissue to reticular dermis is not tight or rigid. Rather, it is loose, allowing the skin a degree of shifting movement over muscle and skeletal structures. The subcutaneous tissue is crisscrossed with connective tissue to fibers and layers interspersed with fat to hold it together. When pockets of fat accumulate between the connective tissue bands beyond the ability of the connective tissue to hold it smooth, the appearance is called *cellulite* or *orange-peel skin*. Because women generally have thinner skin and less rigid connective tissue bands than men, cellulite is generally more apparent in women. It is also more likely to appear in certain areas of the body as well, such as the hips, thighs, and buttocks.

Skin Health Over Time

As children, we take our soft, pliable, quickly healing skin for granted. We play outside, cavort in any available water, and roam hills, valleys, and flats. During this time, our skin is absorbing the effects of this *mild trauma*. The effects are not all bad, but they are certainly cumulative. Every bit of *exposure* has its consequences.

Without question, however, many people get more sun exposure than is necessary for bone health. People who work outside are hard-pressed to avoid the effects of weather, even with generous applications of sunscreen. Even if the sun never touches us, we are bombarded with tiny molecular renegades (radiation) that do their damage. As long as we live, we cannot completely avoid damage to the skin, and it will age.

The **aging** process is both complex and simple. Simply put, it is the degradation of the dermis and epidermis over time that leaves the skin thin, lacking elasticity, lined, and speckled with pigmentation. A reduction in skin turgor occurs.[52] Loss of adhesion between the layers of the epidermis and between the epidermis and dermis create a greater tendency for injury and more visible effects of gravity (wrinkles and folds). Decreases in filaggrin and NMF mean dry and flaky skin. Wound healing slows from a decrease in Langerhans cell production.[53]

To further understand the changes in our skin over time, we use the terms intrinsic aging and extrinsic aging. **Intrinsic aging** occurs by virtue of genetics and gravity—it is unavoidable. **Extrinsic aging** is the portion for which we are responsible. It is aging attributable to external factors such as the sun, pollution, and smoking.

Intrinsic Aging

Because genetics play a noteworthy role in the aging process, some of those effects are out of our hands. The longer we live, the more likely we will face our mother or father in the mirror one day. Intrinsic aging happens over time and regardless of resistance. Clients seen for problems such as deep smile lines or, more typically, vertical upper-lip lines will report that either their mother or father had the same aging symptoms.

Although most of intrinsic aging is out of our control, it does not mean that we should throw up our hands and consider it a lost cause. Advanced skin care techniques, among them microdermabrasion in the clinical setting and sophisticated home care regimes, can blunt the onset of the inevitable.

Extrinsic Aging

Exposure to such environmental hazards as wind, severe temperature changes, sun, smoking, and pollution accelerates the aging process and increases the potential for skin cancers. To the aesthetician, extrinsic aging may be considered the type of aging that we have complete control over. We can protect our skin from extrinsic aging by using sunblock or staying out of the sun altogether. Simply being outside unprotected will age the skin faster. Wind and extremes in temperature will age the skin faster than skin that is not exposed to temperature or wind extremes. An age-controlled comparison of an Iowa farmer's skin to that of a non-gardening suburban mother who shuns the outdoors would reveal a dramatic difference in extrinsic aging.

All clients should be reminded of potential injuries to the skin that occur with extreme or prolonged exposure to the sun, wind, temperature extremes, and pollution. The most significant factor in extrinsic aging is the sun.

Extrinsic aging magnifies **rhytids** (wrinkles), a dull, dry, and sallow appearance of the skin, **actinic keratosis** (overgrowth of skin layers), and irregular pigmentation. Over time, skin that is consistently exposed or has extreme exposure to the environment may develop skin cancers. Although basal cell carcinomas (BCCs) are the most common, more serious squamous cell and melanoma cancers are on the rise. Recent statistics tell the story of decades of sun worship. The American Cancer Society tells us that as of this writing, over 1 million cases of skin cancer have been diagnosed yearly. Most of these cases are considered sun-related. Of the 1 million diagnosed cases each year, over 55,000 of those will be melanoma. Of those diagnosed with melanoma, nearly 10,000 will die.

> A simple yet effective way to manage extrinsic aging is to avoid smoking. It is also thought that secondhand smoke contributes to extrinsic aging. Over time, skin that is consistently exposed or has extreme exposure to the environment may develop skin cancers.

Pigmentary Disorders

Melanin production can increase or decrease beyond normal, creating a mottled appearance in the skin. These problems can be congenital or acquired. It is the responsibility of aestheticians to avoid the latter pitfall in their treatment of clients.

Hyperpigmentation

Hyperpigmentation results from increased deposition of melanin. This irregular pigmentation has origins in solar exposure, pregnancy, medications, and birth control. It can be frustrating, yet is a simple problem to solve.

Hyperpigmentation occurs when melanocytes are over-stimulated in a haphazard fashion. Such is the case in **melasma gravidarum**, commonly known as the *pregnancy mask*. This results not only from pregnancy but also with the use of birth control pills.

Unfortunately, hyperpigmentation can also result from aggressive or mismanaged peeling, microdermabrasion, and intense pulsed light (IPL) therapy (Foto Facial)—from any procedure in which the skin is overstimulated or injured. Hyperpigmentation is especially common in types IV, V, and VI skin.

Hypopigmentation

Hypopigmentation occurs when melanocytes no longer produce melanin, leaving areas of the skin without pigment. Diseases such as vitiligo and leukoderma (in association with inflammatory diseases such as atopic dermatitis) are two relatively common disorders that create hypopigmentation.

Just as with hyperpigmentation, hypopigmentation can also occur when skin has been damaged through aggressive treatment. Any treatment that affects melanocytes may result in hypopigmentation. *White spots* are indicative that melanocytes have been damaged and will no longer produce pigment.

Vitiligo affects approximately 4 percent of the world's population.[54] Affecting the melanocytes of the skin, **vitiligo** causes hypopigmentation that is irreversible. Those afflicted with vitiligo are often psychologically affected and self-conscious of their appearance.

Skin Cancers

Basal Cell Carcinoma

Basal cell carcinoma (BCC) is the most common skin cancer, often found in areas of repeated sunburns and sun exposure (Figure 2–41). A BCC is a slow-growing tumor and generally does not metastasize. It can, however, cause a good deal of disfigurement if left untreated

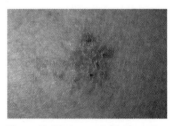

Figure 2–41 An example of superficial BCC. © Milady, a part of Cengage Learning

or treated ineffectually. In the United States, the incidence of BCC annually is nearly 900,000 (550,000 men and 350,000 women).[55] Six subtypes of BCC exist: (1) nodular, (2) pigmented, (3) superficial, (4) micronodular, (5) cystic, and (6) morpheaform. Each subset has its own distinct features. The most common appearance of BCC is as a pearly nodule. It can exhibit some but not necessarily all of the following features: bleeding, crusting, and a small center depression.

Squamous Cell Carcinoma

Squamous cell carcinoma (SCC) is the second most common skin cancer, with over 200,000 cases diagnosed annually[56] (Figure 2–42). Unlike BCC, SCC can sometimes metastasize if left untreated. As with BCC, chronic sun exposure seems to be the main precursor to SCC, although it has been found in areas without sun exposure, such as the mucous membranes

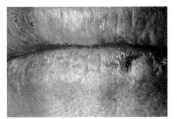

Figure 2–42 An example of squamous cell carcinoma. © Milady, a part of Cengage Learning

of the mouth. Usually, areas such as the inside of the mouth have been exposed to frequent and persistent sores, such as leukoplakia. On a rare occasion, SCC will spring up in an area of healthy skin. The hypothesis is that SCC may be passed genetically.

Melanoma

Melanoma is the most dangerous of all skin cancers because it will metastasize and can cause death (Figure 2–43). It is important that you are always alert to the potential for melanoma. Melanoma is an irregularly shaped and irregularly colored mole, most commonly occurring on the back of the legs and trunk. Those who have had one to two significant sunburns are at risk for melanoma. Because these moles are not primarily located on the face, it is important for the aesthetician to be an *investigator*, asking the client about moles that are new or have changed. You can never be too careful when you suspect a melanoma and should refer the client to a physician. Remember the ABCDs of skin cancer, and you could save a life!

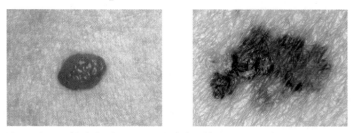

Figure 2–43 This lesion is asymmetrical; the sides are uneven. © Milady, a part of Cengage Learning

ABCDs of Cancer

Asymmetry—Growth that, when divided in half, has two mismatched halves.

Border irregularity—Ragged or uneven edges that are blurred and poorly defined.

Color—Uneven black, brown, and tan coloring; other colors, like red, white, and blue, can also be interspersed in the growth; any change in the color of the preexisting mole or lesion.

Diameter—Any growth larger than the top of a pencil eraser, which is approximately 6 millimeters in diameter; any unusual or sudden increase in size should also be checked.

Conclusion

On the surface, the skin looks like an uncomplicated structure, simply meant to protect our inner organs from injury. However, as you can see, the skin is extraordinarily complex. Many cells work to keep the skin healthy and free from infection or disease. Without a doubt you will return to this chapter and continue to expand your knowledge of the skin as you build your medical aesthetics career.

Chapter References

1. Gray, J. (1997). *The world of skin care.* Available online at http://www.pg.com.
2. Spense, A. P. (2004, February 22). *Basic human anatomy* (3rd ed.). Available online at http://www.sawyerproducts.com.

3. Nemours Foundation. (2004). *Skin, hair, and nails.* Available online at http://www.kidshealth.org.
4. American Society of Plastic Surgeons. (2003, December). *2002 Quick facts on cosmetic and reconstructive surgery trends.* Available online at http://www.plasticsurgery.org.
5. Merck & Co. (2001). *Resource library.* Available online at http://www.mercksource.com.
6. Ganong, W. F. (1989). Initiation of impulses in sense organs. In *Review of medical physiology* (14th ed.). Norwalk, CT: Appleton & Lange.
7. Merck & Co. (2001). *Resource library.* Available online at http://www.mercksource.com.
8. Students of Elert, G. (2001). *Temperature of a healthy human (skin temperature).* Available online at http://hypertextbook.com.
9. Nova. (2000, November). *Surviving Denali.* Available online at http://www.pbs.org
10. Gray, J. (1997). *The world of skin care.* Available online at http://www.pg.com/.
11. Gray, J. (1997). *The world of skin care.* Available online at http://www.pg.com.
12. Gray, J. (1997). *The world of skin care.* Available online at http://www.pg.com.
13. Gray, J. (1997). *The world of skin care.* Available online at http://www.pg.com.
14. Nemours Foundation. (2004). *Skin, hair, and nails.* Available online at http://www.kidshealth.org.
15. Nemours Foundation. (2004). *Skin, hair, and nails.* Available online at http://www.kidshealth.org.
16. University of Iowa Healthcare. (2004, March 15). *Fluid replacement.* Available online at http://www.uihealthcare.com.
17. Elsner, P., & Maibach, H. L. (2000). *Cosmeceuticals: Drugs vs. cosmetics.* New York: Marcel Dekker.
18. Gray, J. (1997). *The world of skin care.* Available online at http://www.pg.com.
19. eMedicine.com, Inc. (2004). *Hair growth.* Available online at http://www.emedicine.com.
20. Nemours Foundation. (2004). *Skin, hair, and nails.* Available online at http://www.kidshealth.org.
21. Gray, J. (1997). *The world of skin care.* Available online at http://www.pg.com.
22. King, D. (2003, November 14). *Introduction to skin histology.* Available online at http://www.Siumed.edu.
23. Spense, A. P. (2004, February 22). *Basic human anatomy* (3rd ed.). Available online at http://www.sawyerproducts.com.
24. King, D. (2003, November 14). *Introduction to skin histology.* Available online at http://www.Siumed.edu.

25. Lowe, N., & Sellar, P. (1999). *Skin secrets: The medical facts versus the beauty fiction.* New York: Collins & Brown.
26. Baumann, L. (2002). *Cosmetic dermatology practices and principles.* New York: McGraw-Hill.
27. Baumann, L. (2002). *Cosmetic dermatology practices and principles.* New York: McGraw-Hill.
28. King, D. (2003, November 14). *Introduction to skin histology.* Available online at http://www.Siumed.edu.
29. King, D. (2003, November 14). *Introduction to skin histology.* Available online at http://www.Siumed.edu.
30. King, D. (2003, November 14). *Introduction to skin histology.* Available online at http://www.Siumed.edu.
31. Spense, A. P. (2004, February 22). *Basic human anatomy* (3rd ed.). Available online at http://www.sawyerproducts.com.
32. Moschella, S., Pillsbury, D., & Hurley, H. (1975). *Dermatology* (Vol. 1). Philadelphia: W. B. Saunders Company.
33. King, D. (2003, November 14). *Introduction to skin histology.* Available online at http://www.Siumed.edu.
34. King, D. (2003, November 14). *Introduction to skin histology.* Available online at http://www.Siumed.edu.
35. King, D. (2003, November 14). *Introduction to skin histology.* Available online at http://www.Siumed.edu.
36. Shea, C., & Prieto, V. G. (2003, October 13). *Merkel cell carcinoma.* Available online at http://www.emedicine.com.
37. Baumann, L. (2002). *Cosmetic dermatology practices and principles.* New York: McGraw-Hill.
38. King, D. (2003, November 14). *Introduction to skin histology.* Available online at http://www.Siumed.edu.
39. Spense, A. P. (2004, February 22). *Basic human anatomy* (3rd ed.). Available online at http://www.sawyerproducts.com.
40. King, D. (2003, November 14). *Introduction to skin histology.* Available online at http://www.Siumed.edu.
41. King, D. (2003, November 14). *Introduction to skin histology.* Available online at http://www.Siumed.edu.
42. Nemours Foundation. (2004). *Skin, hair, and nails.* Available online at http://www.kidshealth.org.
43. Spense, A. P. (2004, February 22). *Basic human anatomy* (3rd ed.). Available online at http://www.sawyerproducts.com.
44. Obagi, Z. (2002). *Skin health restoration and rejuvenation.* New York: Springer-Verlag.
45. Baumann, L. (2002). *Cosmetic dermatology practices and principles.* New York: McGraw-Hill.
46. King, D. (2003, November 14). *Introduction to skin histology.* Available online at http://www.Siumed.edu.

47. Spense, A. P. (2004, February 22). *Basic human anatomy* (3rd ed.). Available online at http://www.sawyerproducts.com.
48. King, D. (2003, November 14). *Introduction to skin histology.* Available online at http://www.Siumed.edu.
49. King, D. (2003, November 14). *Introduction to skin histology.* Available online at http://www.Siumed.edu.
50. King, D. (2003, November 14). *Introduction to skin histology.* Available online at http://www.Siumed.edu.
51. Nemours Foundation. (2004). *Skin, hair, and nails.* Available online at http://www.kidshealth.org.
52. Obagi, Z. (2002). *Skin health restoration and rejuvenation.* New York: Springer-Verlag.
53. Bisaccia, E., & Scarborough, D. (2002). *The Columbia manual of dermatologic cosmetic surgery.* New York: McGraw-Hill.
54. Parsad, D., Sunil, D., & Kanwar, A. J. (2003, October 23). Quality of life in clients with vitiligo. *Journal of Health and Quality of Life Outcomes,* 1(1):58.
55. Revis, Jr., D. R. (2001, July). *Skin grafts, split thickness.* Available online at http://www.emedicine.com.
56. The Skin Cancer Foundation. (2004). *About squamous cell.* Available online at http://www.skincancer.org.

Bibliography

Boone, T. (2003). Why is anatomy important? http://faculty.css.edu/tboone2/asep/Anatomy.html.

Marieb, E. N. (2006). *Essentials of human anatomy and physiology,* San Francisco: Pearson Benjamin Cummings.

Medical Terminology

A Brief History of Medical Terminology

When early physicians were first identifying anatomical structures, abnormalities, and functions, they realized a need to have an organized classification system. With so many words being added to the lexicon, it became necessary to set in place a formalized, structured methodology for the nomenclature. Since doctors were scattered across a wide geographic area and communication was slow and unreliable, early doctors needed to implement a system that would prevent things from being named multiple times, or named inconsistently. The father of medical terminology is the father of modern medicine himself, Hippocrates. Understanding how medical terminology has evolved over the centuries will help to make sense of the words that you will begin to use every day.

Egyptian, Greek, and Roman Influences

One of the first recorded physicians to use medical terminology to describe diseases or medical conditions was **Hippocrates**. The "father of medical terminology," as he might also be referred to, is credited with the *Hippocratic Corpus*, a collection of more than 60 early medical works on diseases, genealogy, and other assorted medical subjects. Hippocrates was quite brilliant in his forethought to make the language of medicine universal. To accomplish this, the father of modern medicine referred to the texts left behind by Imhotep.

Though he is most known as the architect responsible for building the first of Egypt's pyramids, Imhotep is also considered one of the world's first physicians. Many believe that Imhotep was the writer of the *Edwin Smith Papyrus*, one of the oldest surviving pieces of medical literature. The papyrus, a medical treatise that describes 48 injuries, using more than 90 medical terms, is thought by others to have been written by a minimum of three different authors. Whoever the writer of the papyrus, the knowledge that was gathered in it served as a starting point for Greek and Roman terms, most of which had previously been based on mythology, legend, and physical descriptions. The knowledge that Imhotep passed on to his protégés was fine-tuned and adopted by the Romans.

At the time, most Greek and Roman medical terms were based on mythology, legend, and physical description. Since most of these myths and legends were meant to explain the unexplainable, the remnants of these words left in medical terminology are often amusing. For example, in Homer's myth, the *Odyssey*, drinking from the River Lethe leads to fatigue and sluggishness, or **lethargy**.[1] Legends have also made permanent marks in the medical lexicon. The terms *atlas*, *Achilles' heel*, and *cancer* all have origins in legends of the day.[2]

However, prior to the implementation of universal terminology, most terms were coined using physical descriptions. *Kyposis* (hump-back) is an example of this. Legends have also made permanent marks in the medical lexicon. For example, the *atlas*, or first cervical vertebra, is named for Atlas, the Greek god of legend who supported the world on his shoulders. The naming of disorders based on clinical descriptions was used routinely for the next few centuries.

The Middle Ages and Renaissance Period

The coining of terms in the Middle Ages, like that of the Greeks and Romans, relied on clinical descriptions, even though they were often medically—and politically—incorrect. A term from this period is *clubfoot*, a disorder so named because of the sound the deformed foot made on medieval castle floors.

One of the defining characteristics of the Middle Ages and Renaissance period was an increase in intercontinental travel afforded by advancements in shipbuilding and cartography. This perpetuated a similar intercontinental influence on medical terminology, causing cross-cultural hybrids of words to appear. For example, the term *orthopedics* is a combination of the Latin *ortho* (straight) and the Greek *paedic* (child).

Further complicating matters, religious influences made their way into the lexicon we still use today. When we aren't feeling well, we say that we are "sick." That word is thought to originate from the Old English *sucan,* or the sucking of the devil at one's soul.[3]

Contemporary Times

Medical terminology as it has come to be hit its stride in concurrence with medical advancements themselves. Advancements in pharmacology, diagnosis, and disease pathology had their renaissance during the later part of the nineteenth and early twentieth centuries. During this time, words were added to the lexicon with fervent speed. Since then, the medical community has organized to renovate prior mistakes and inaccuracies in nomenclature. Organizations and individuals have and are constantly seeking out misnomers and other errors in the medical terminology. Often, several names for one item are retired and one name is accepted in accordance with the goals of medicine. Chief among the goals of modern medical terminology is the elimination of words that carry judgment or reflect opinions toward affected populations.

How Medical Terminology is Used in the Aesthetic Environment

While certain guidelines may be set forth, there are many facets of medical terminology that make learning it difficult and taxing. There is no one-way, suits-all way for someone to learn this specialized language. Especially for aestheticians in training, the degree to which they understand and use it will be limited and dependent upon local circumstances. While in-depth understanding of word analysis—dissecting a word to ascertain its meaning—is appropriate, in-depth studies and rote memorization of specific terms are not.

However, by learning the meaning of common Greek or Latin root words, you can understand the meaning of most medical terms based on them. The use of suffixes and prefixes gives further clarity. For example, the root *nephr* means pertaining to the kidneys. The suffix -*ology* means the study of something. Therefore, nephrology would be the study of the kidneys.

By being consistent and learned in the area of medical terminology, you will be able to decipher the meaning of words, even if you haven't heard of or seen the word itself before. As an aesthetician you may, for example, run across the word dermatitis. While you may know it is skin that itches or has a rash, it may be more interesting to know that the exact meaning of **dermatitis** is skin inflammation.

As an aesthetician, you know that *derma* refers to an inner layer of the skin. Because you know that, you can deduce that *dermatitis* is a skin inflammation, that *dermatology* is the study of the skin, and that *dermoplasty* is the repair of the skin. As you can see from this very simple example, knowing and understanding medical root words can be of assistance in defining some unfamiliar medical terms.

> Medical terminology includes eponyms, in which a treatment or disorder is named after the founder or first recorded case. Examples of this include Dercum's disease, named for Francis X. Dercum, a U.S. neurologist; Alzheimer's disease, named for Alois Alzheimer, a German neurologist; and Lou Gehrig's disease, named for the professional baseball player known to have suffered the disease.[4] Unfortunately, there is no easy way to learn eponyms.

Word Analysis

Now that we have examined some of the broader fundamentals associated with medical terminology, you should be ready to begin the process of learning about the words themselves and some of the basics and exceptions that make medical terminology so complex.

Medical terminology is much like a puzzle. By using word analysis, and dissecting a word, you can isolate the different parts of a word, and unlock the puzzle. Once you can isolate the different parts of a word and define them, you can use this knowledge to help define many other pertinent words.

When examining a medical term, begin at the end of the word, or the suffix, and then go back to the beginning. To best find the suffix, isolate the different parts of the word. Look for the "o," or another combining vowel. The root word plus the combining vowel is the combining form. Let's use the word *mammography*:

MAMM/ O /   GRAPHY
Combining Form   Suffix

Sometimes, a medical term will have more than one root word. Since the combining vowel connects the root word to the suffix, you will most often find a corresponding number of combining forms in this case.[5]

In many cases, there will be a prefix before the combining from. A prefix modifies the root word, usually quantifying or qualifying it. For example, *intravenous* breaks down to *within a vein*.

Note that not all words are structured in the same format. Take note that in the word *intravenous* there is no combining vowel. When the suffix begins with a vowel, as is the case with *-ous,* the combining vowel is dropped. Once you've established the suffix, you are ready to move on to the root word, the most important part of a medical term.

Root Words

The root is the most basic component of a word, and it is the basis for which the meaning of a word is constructed. Often, roots can stand alone, as is the case with *graph, cycl(e), pyr(e), crypt*, and *term*. Most roots in medical terminology, however, do need other components. A word can contain more than one root (Table 3–1).

TABLE 3–1 Common Root Words Found in the Aesthetic Environment

Root Word	Meaning	Origin	Example	Meaning
ADIP-	fat	Latin	*adipocele*	a hernia with a hernial sac
			adiposis	obesity, either local or widespread
ANDR-	male	Greek	*andromorphous*	having the shape or structure of man
			adrogenic	pertaining to males

TABLE 3–1 (continued)

Root Word	Meaning	Origin	Example	Meaning
ANTH-	flower	Greek	*exanthema*	an eruption outside the body or on the skin
ARC-	arched	Latin	*arciform*	shaped like an arch
BLEPHAR-	eyelid	Greek	*blepharoplasty*	cosmetic or corrective surgery on the eyelid
BULL-	blister	Latin	*bulla*	lymph-filled blister, usually within the epidermis
CARCIN-	Cancer	Greek	*carcinogen*	any substance known or thought to cause cancer
			carcinoma	malignant skin tumor
CALL-	hardened skin	Latin	*callous*	pertaining to a localized area of hard skin
CAPILL-	hair	Greek	*capillo-venous*	the meeting point of a venule and a capillary
			capilliculture	hair-loss treatment
CAU-	to burn	Greek	*cauterize*	use of an agent or instrument to burn tissue
CHEIL-; CHIL-	lip	Greek	*acheilia*	congenital absence of the lips
			cheiloplasty	corrective or plastic surgery on the lips
CHIR-	hand	Greek	*chiroplasty*	any cosmetic or corrective surgery on the hands
CHROM-; CHROMAT-	color	Greek	*chromatin*	photosensitive substance within the cells that change color

TABLE 3–1 (continued)

Root Word	Meaning	Origin	Example	Meaning
COLL(A)-	glue	Greek	*collagen*	protein found in connective tissue
CORN-	horny	Latin	*cornification*	tissue deterioration into dead horny tissue
			subcorneous	beneath the horny layer
CRINE-	to secrete	Greek	*endocrine*	excreted internally
			exocrine	excreted externally
			neurocrine	secreted from newer cells
CUT-	skin	Latin	*intracutaneous*	within the skin
			cutin	found in upper epidermis
CYST-	bladder; cyst	Greek	*cystitis*	inflammation of the bladder
			hematocyst	a blood-filled cyst
			polycystic	many cysts
DERM-; DERMAT-	skin	Greek	*dermatophyte*	group of fungi that reside underneath the skin and appendages
			dermographia	condition in which the skin is particularly susceptible to irritation
			mesoderm	layer of skin that houses connective tissue and muscles
EDE-	to swell	Greek	*edema*	swelling due to fluid accumulation within tissue
ERYTHR-	red	Greek	*erythroderma*	condition characterized by redness of the skin

TABLE 3–1 (continued)

Root Word	Meaning	Origin	Example	Meaning
FIBR-	fiber	Latin	*fibril*	a small component of the larger fiber
			fibrin	a protein that plays a role in blood clotting
FOLL-	bag	Latin	*follicle*	a small sac with secretory functions
			folliculitis	inflammation of a follicle
GLAB(R)-	smooth	Latin	*glabella*	the region on the forehead between the eyebrows
HEM-; HEMAT-	blood	Greek	*hematobic*	living in the blood
			hematocrit	centrifuge used to separate blood cells
			hemolytic	the destruction of red blood cells
HEPAT-, HEPAR-	liver	Greek	*heparin*	substance in the liver that can prolong blood clotting
HIST-; HISTI-	tissue	Greek	*histokinesis*	study of the activity of the smallest known structures of the body
KER-; KERAT-	horny tissue	Greek	*keratinization*	development of horny tissue
LACRIM-	tear	Latin	*lacrimal*	pertaining to tears or tear ducts
			nasolacrimal	pertaining to the tear-producing organs and the nose
LATER-	side	Latin	*lateral*	pertaining to the side
			dorsolateral	pertaining to the side and the back
			heterolateral	pertaining to the opposite side
			bilateral	pertaining to both sides

TABLE 3–1 (continued)

Root Word	Meaning	Origin	Example	Meaning
LEPT-	delicate	Greek	*leptodermatous*	thin-skinned
LIP-	fat	Greek	*lipodystrophy*	condition characterized by the elimination of fat in certain parts of the body, but not others
			lipolysis	destruction of fat and fat cells
LUM-	light	Latin	*lumen*	the inner portion of a tubular structure
			luminosity	ability to emit light
LYMPH-	pertaining to the lymphs	Greek	*lymphoderma*	effecting the lymphatics of the skin
MACUL-	spot	Latin	*macula*	a spot of discoloration
			emaculation	removal of freckles and spots, including skin tumors
			maculopapular	pertaining to a spot and a papule
MAL-	cheek	Latin	*malar*	pertaining to the cheek
			maloplasty	corrective or plastic surgery on the cheeks or cheekbones
MELAN-	dark	Greek	*melanin*	dark brown pigment
			melanism	abnormal pigmentation of tissue
			melanoderma	dark mispigmentation of the skin

TABLE 3–1 (continued)

Root Word	Meaning	Origin	Example	Meaning
MORPH-	to form or to change	Greek	morphology	the study of structure and form
			dysmorphophobia	fear of deformation
			anamorphosis	gradual evolution from one form to another
NAR-	nostril	Latin	nariform	shaped as a nostril
NECR-	dead tissue	Greek	necrosis	pertaining to dead tissue
NERV-	nerve	Latin	innervation	the placement and distribution of nerves
			abnerval	positioned away from a nerve
OCUL-	pertaining to the eye	Latin	oculomotor	pertaining to the functions that cause the eyeball to move
			binocular	vision with the use of two eyes
OP-; OPT-	eye	Greek	myopia	nearsighted
			optician	person who makes corrective eyewear
OPTHALM-	pertaining to the eye	Greek	xeropthalmia	condition in which the conjunctiva is dry and hardened
			exophthalmic	abnormal protrusion of the eyeball from its socket
			ophthal-mologist	person who specializes in the treatment of disorders affecting the eye

TABLE 3-1 (continued)

Root Word	Meaning	Origin	Example	Meaning
OT-	ear	Greek	*diotic*	both ears
			parotid	situated near the ear
PATH-	disease or feeling	Greek	*idiopathic*	disease for which there is no known cause
			pathology	the study of disease
PELL-	skin	Latin	*pellicle*	a sheer, protective coating of skin
PIL-	hair	Latin	*pilosebaceous*	pertaining to the hair follicles and accompanying sebum-secreting glands
			pilose	high hair density
			pilocystic	hair- and fat-encysted tumors
			epilate	to remove a hair from the root, causing damage to the follicle
PHLEB-	vein	Greek	*phlebismus*	inflammation of the vein
			phleboclysis	the use of saline to flush a vein
PHOT-	light	Greek	*photolytic*	able to be decomposed with light
PLAS(T)-	to form or mold	Greek	*hyperplasia*	excessive tissue formation due to increased cell production
			rhinoplasty	plastic surgery done to reshape the tissue in or around the nose
RHIN-; RHINE-	nose	Greek	*rhinoplasty*	plastic surgery done to reshape the tissue in or around the nose

TABLE 3–1 (continued)

Root Word	Meaning	Origin	Example	Meaning
SARC-	flesh	Greek	*sarcobionic*	living on skin
			sarcoma	malignant tumor on connective tissues
SCLER-	hardened	Greek	*sclera*	the fibrous outer coating of the eyeball
THERM-	heat	Greek	*hyperthermaglasia*	sensitivity to heat
			hypothermia	dangerously low body temperature
TOX-	poison	Greek	*cytotoxin*	cell poisoning substance found in blood serum
			toxidermatitis	skin inflammation as a result of poisoning
			antitoxin	any substance that can counteract the effects of poisoning
			toxicology	the study of poisons and their effects on the body
TRICH-	hair	Greek	*melantrichous*	dark–haired
TROPH-	development		*autotroph*	capable of self-nourishment
			hypertrophy	size increase independent of normal growth
			dystrophy	inadequate or compromised nutrition

Suffixes

Knowing the Greek and Latin origin of a word's suffix can help us determine the meaning. Prefixes modify their root words by indicating whether the word is a noun, an adjective, plural, or diminutive (Table 3–2).

TABLE 3–2 Common Suffixes Found in Aesthetic Environments

Adjective Endings	Meaning	Examples
-ac, -al, -ary, -ic, -ical, -ous, -tic, -ar	—	cardiac, skeletal, salivary, pelvic, surgical, venous, paralytic, muscular
Noun Endings		
-iac	indicates person afflicted with certain diseases or conditions	hemophiliac
-ia	an unhealthy state, condition of	anesthesia
-is	with, having the nature/condition of	cutis
-ism	condition, state of being	alcoholism
-ist	one who specializes	radiologist
-itis	inflammation	arthritis
-logy	study of	biology
-plasty	surgical repair of	rhinoplasty
-oma	tumor or mass	carcinoma
-scopy	process of examination	laproscopy
-pathy	disease, suffering	neuropathy
-gen	producing/forming	pathogen
Diminutive Endings		
-ole	—	arteriole
-icle	small, little, minute	particle
-ule	small, little, minute	venule

Suffixes help us determine the meaning of a word by describing the use of the word in question. It tells us if the word is a noun or nouns, whether it describes something, or its relationship to something else.

Prefixes

Knowing the Greek and Latin roots of a word's prefix can also help us determine the meaning of the word. As mentioned earlier, prefixes modify the root words by either qualifying or quantifying them. Quantity can be determined by using the prefix *poly-* to designate a general number, or by using a specific number, as is the case with *tri-*. Quantity can also be designated as a negation, like *in-* or *im-,* meaning without.

Prefixes can also qualify the root in terms of time or direction. *Ante*, for instance, means before, and if we connect it with *mortem* we end up with *antemortem*, or prior to death.

Most often, Greek prefixes are attached to words that will modify or change their original meanings. Originally, many prefixes stood alone as prepositions or adverbs. However, they rarely stand alone anymore.[6] Prefixes often end in a vowel, though the vowel is dropped when the root word ends in an *h*, or another vowel (see Table 3–3).

TABLE 3–3 **Common Prefixes Used in the Aesthetic Environment**

Prefix	Meaning	Origin	Example	Meaning
A-, AB-, ABS-	from	Latin	*abnormal*	deviating from that which would otherwise be expected under a given set of circumstances
			abarthrosis	condition in which bones rub against one another
AD-, AC-, AG-, AL-	near, to, or toward	Latin	*Adrenal*	near the kidneys
			aggressive	a course of progression that is more rapid or recurrent than would otherwise be expected
			alleviate	any mechanism that remedies a symptom or symptoms

TABLE 3–3 (continued)

Prefix	Meaning	Origin	Example	Mean ing
ANTI-	opposite	Greek	*antipruritic*	anything that relieves an itch
			antibiotic	relationship between two organisms in which one will kill the other
CIRCUM-	around	Latin	*circumference*	the distance around
			circumvent	to take a path that intentionally avoids a sensitive area
COM-; CON-; CO-	with	Latin	*complicate*	to fold
			conjunctiva	mucous membrane that lines the eyelid
DYS-	bad or difficult	Greek	*dystrophy*	inadequate or compromised nutrition
ENDO-; ENTO-	within	Greek	*endocrine*	excreted internally
EPI-	upon	Greek	*epidemic*	a disease that is rampant on a localized level
			epidermis	layer of skin
HYPER-	more	Greek	*hypergia*	an increase in functional activity
			hyperergy	sensitivity to allergens
HYPO-	less	Greek	*hypogastropagus*	conjoined twins, joined at the stomach region
			hypophrenia	having or relating to feeblemindedness
IM-; IN-	into	Latin	*insult*	any event that causes the discontinuation of a tissue
			inappetence	loss of desire
			impalpable	unable to be detected by touch

TABLE 3–3 (continued)

Prefix	Meaning	Origin	Example	Meaning
INTRA-; INTRO-	within	Latin	*intraocular*	within the eye cavity
			intravenous	inside the veins
			introcession	a depression or dip in the surface
PER-	through or wrongly	Latin	*percussion*	to firmly tap the body to use the vibratory effects as a means of diagnosis
			perfusion	the movement of fluid through a certain space
PERI-	around or nearby	Greek	*peripheral*	related to, located in, or constituting an outer boundary
			pericranium	the outer surface of the cranial bones
PRO-	before	Greek	*progeria*	premature senility
			prognosis	an educated guess as to cause, course, and treatment of a given set of symptoms
PRE-	before	Latin	*prescription*	authorization for a patient to use a controlled substance for therapeutic purposes
			preclusion	inability to perform movement
POST-	after or behind	Latin	*postcardial*	positioned at the rear of the heart or behind the heart
			postmortem	after death
			postnasal	occurring behind the nose

TABLE 3–3 (continued)

Prefix	Meaning	Origin	Example	Meaning
PRO-	forward or in front	Latin	*prognosis*	an educated guess as to cause, course, and treatment of a given set of symptoms
			proliferate	to grow with multiplicity
			projectile	to cast away with speed and distance
RE-; RED-	again	Latin	*resection*	the process of cutting out, as in a growth
			respiration	the act of taking in oxygen, and circulating it around the body while removing carbon dioxide
RETRO-	backwards or back	Latin	*retrography*	condition characterized by writing backwards
			retronasal	positioned in the rear of the nasal cavity
SE-	away	Latin	*secernment*	glandular secretion
			secrete	to expel outward or discharge
SUB-; SUC-; SUF-; SUP-	under or somewhat	Latin	*subapical*	near the top
			subaqueous	below water
			succursale	secondary part to a greater whole
			suffusion	the spreading of fluid in a given space
			suppository	medication in the form of a soft solid, administered by placement in an orifice

TABLE 3–3 (continued)

Prefix	Meaning	Origin	Example	Meaning
SUPER-; SUPRA-	above	Latin	*superscription*	the R$_x$ at the beginning of a prescription
SYM-	with or together	Greek	*asymmetrical*	two sides that are not equal
			symbiosis	the union of two organisms for mutual benefit
TRANS-; TRAN-; TRA-	across	Latin	*translucid*	opaque to transparent
			transverse	to position in the form of a cross
ULTRA-	beyond	Latin	*ultrasound*	the use of sound waves as a mechanism for diagnosis
			ultrastructure	a grouping of minute particles in an organized fashion

Like Greek prefixes, prefixes derived from Latin are added to other words to change or modify their meanings. Most Latin prefixes are Latin words from which the traditional Latin ending (-*a*, -*um*, and -*is*) has been removed. For example, the Latin word *finis* means "end." The -*is* ending is dropped, and we see the Latin base *fin* in such English words as "final." Latin prefixes, like Greek prefixes, are often used together with Greek root words. This means that many words can have a Latin prefix with a Greek root, or vice versa. Similarly, a root word may be preceded by any number of prefixes, which all collaborate with one another toward the goal of changing and modifying the root.

Plurals

As you know, the plurals of many words in the English language are often difficult to ascertain. In some instances, the words are completely different (mouse/mice) or they are the same as the singular (deer/deer). A similar challenge exists for those in the medical communities. Some might argue that the use of proper plurals can be one of the more challenging aspects of medical terminology. The problem is so pervasive that even a lot of physicians experience difficulty with them.

While difficult, plurals generally follow some basic rules.[7] By taking the time to learn these rules, you will be prepared to tackle these challenges when they do arise.

The following table (Table 3–4) is meant to provide some of the more common rules of forming plurals.

TABLE 3–4 Basic Rules for Forming Medical Plurals[8]

If the Singular Ending Is	Singular Example	The Plural Rule Is	Plural Form
-is	diagnosis	Drop the -is and add -es	diagnoses
-um	ileum	Drop the -um and add -a	ilea
-us	alveolus	Drop the -us and add -i	alveoli
-a	vertebra	Drop the -a and add -ae	vertebrae
-ix	appendix	Drop the -ix and add -ices	appendices
-ex	cortex	Drop the -ex and add -ices	cortices
-ex	thorax	Drop the -x and add -ces	thoraces
-ma	sarcoma	Retain the -ma and add -ta	sarcomata
-on	spermatozoon	Drop the -on and add -a	spermatozoa
-nx	larynx	Drop the -x and add -ges	larynges
-y	deformity	Drop the -y and add -ies	deformities
-yx	calyx	Drop the -yx and add -yces	calyces
-en	foramen	Drop the -en and add -ina	foramina

However, every rule has an exception. But they are rare, as explained below.

Ten Common Exceptions to Basic Plural Rules[9]:

1. Sometimes the proper plural of a word ending in *-is* will be formed by dropping the *-is* and adding *-ides*. For example, *epididymis* becomes *epididymides*.

2. Sometimes the proper plural of a word ending in *-us* will be formed by dropping the *-us* and adding *-era* or *-ora*. For example: *viscus* becomes *viscera*; *corpus* becomes *corpora*.

3. Some words ending in *-ix* or *-ax* have more than one acceptable plural form. For example: The plural of *appendix* can be either *appendices* or *appendixes*—although the most common plural form would utilize the *-ices* ending.

4. The proper plural for certain words ending in *-ion* can be formed simply by adding an *s*. For example: *chorion* becomes *chorions*.

5. The plural form of the term *vas* is *vasa*.

6. The plural form of *pons* is *pontes*.

7. The plural form of the dual-meaning word *os* is *ora* when referring to mouths and *ossa* when referring to bones.

8. The plural form of the term *femur* is *femora*.

9. The plural form of *cornu* is *cornua*.

10. The plural form of *paries* is *parietes*.

Pronunciation

Pronunciation is a fundamental, yet key concept for anyone in the medical fields. Regardless of the vast wealth of knowledge a person's head may contain, it will be difficult to view the person as credible unless he or she pronounces the vernácular with precision. In medical terminology, many words are long and complicated. They are rather easy to mispronounce. Any professional who intends to work with patients or other medical personnel must have a grasp on pronunciation, which requires both patience and diligence. The dictionary that follows contains pronunciation keys for most terms, but it is also helpful to know the following guidelines.

Words that have the following combination of letters at the beginning of the word are often pronounced in the following ways (Table 3–5):

TABLE 3–5 **Silent Letters**[10]

Letter Combination	Sound	Example	Pronunciation
pt	t	pterygoid	**TEHR**-ih-goyd
ps	s	psoriasis	soh-**RYE**-uh-sis
pn	n	pneometer	nee-**AHM**-uh-ter
gn	n	gnathitis	nuh-**THYE**-tis
mn	n	mnemonic	nuh-**MOHN**-ik

If a prefix ending in a vowel comes before the following combination of letters, then the first letter is pronounced:

hemoptysis-	hee-**MOP**-tih-sis
prognathism-	**PROHG**-nuh-tizm
polypnea-	pohl-**IHP**-nee-uh
dysgnathia-	dihs-**NAH**-thee-uh

Combination of vowels—*oe* and *ae* (British English spelling)—are pronounced as *-ee*. *Ce/cae/coe* are pronounced as *see* and *ge/gae/goe* as "*jee*" in English.

haema	**HEE**-muh
rugae	roo-**JEE**
coelum	**SEE**-luhm
septicaemia	**sehp**-tuh-**SEE**-mee-uh
caecum	**SEE**-kuhm

Additional combinations of letters are pronounced as follows[11]:

Letter Combination	Sound	Word	Pronunciation
ph	f	phrenoplegia	**freh**-noh-**PLEE**-jee-uh
rh	r	rhytidosis	rye-tih-**DOH**-sis
ch	k	cochlea	**COAK**-lee-uh
x	z	xanthic	**ZAN**-thik
dys	dis	dysphagia	dis-**FAY**-jee-uh

There are always exceptions to the rule, of course. But the general guidelines provided can be considered a good starting point when figuring out how to pronounce a new term.

Conclusion

Working in the medispa environment can seem intimidating at first. The expectations and the people, as well as the vernacular, are quite different from a resort or day spa. The clients and the staff will hold you to a higher level of performance, understanding, and professionalism. It is not for the weak of spirit.

Certainly one of the best means of matriculating into this environment is by having a firm grasp of medical terminology. Rote memorization is one way to do this, but if you are able to dissect and use complex medical terms when talking to your peers and explaining these terms to your clients you will go far in the medispa environment.

Just remember—as an aesthetician, your goal is to work hand-in-hand with your clients to realize their skin care goals, not to impress or overwhelm them with words. That being the case, your usage of medical terminology may be somewhat limited, but your ability to understand it is not.

Chapter References

1. Bailey, J.A. *The black voice news.* http://www.blackvoices.com.
2. Bailey, J.A. *The black voice news.* http://www.blackvoices.com.
3. Klein, Ernest. *A comprehensive etymological dictionary of the English language: Dealing with the origin of words and their sense development thus illustrating the history of civilization and culture.* A-K. New York: Elsevier, 1966.
4. Thomas, M.D., M.P.H., C. L. (Ed.). (1997). *Taber's cyclopedic medical dictionary* (Vol. 18). Philadelphia, PA: F. A. Davis.
5. Chabner, D.E. *Medical terminology: A short course.*
6. Bioscientific Terminology.
7. MTWorld.com. "Medical Plurals." http://www.mtworld.com/tools_resources/medical_plurals.html.
8. MTWorld.com. "Medical Plurals." http://www.mtworld.com/tools_resources/medical_plurals.html.
9. MTWorld.com. "Medical Plurals." http://www.mtworld.com/tools_resources/medical_plurals.html.
10. The Medical Terminology Web site of the English Centre. "Pronunciation of Some Medical Words." http://ec.hku.hk/mt/pronunciation.htm
11. The Medical Terminology Web site of the English Centre. "Pronunciation of Some Medical Words." http://ec.hku.hk/mt/pronunciation.htm

Dictionary of Terms

Those terms not easily pronounced based on intuition, phonetics, or common knowledge have a "sounds-like" pronunciation set in parentheses following the term. Those terms are essentially respelled in syllables common to the English language, or forms that are easily recognizable.

Pronounce the terms as they appear in the parentheses. The strongest, or primary, accented syllable is set in boldface and capital letters. The secondary accented syllable is set in boldface and lowercase letters.

5-aminolevulenic (uh-meen-oh-lev-yoo-LINE-ik) **acid (ALA)—** 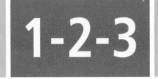 photosensensitizing agent that contains a 20% solution of hydrochloride salt of aminolevulenic acid; for example, Levulan Kerastick. ALA is a metabolic precursor to the photosensitizer PpIX. Used topically to enhance light absorption into the skin. Used most commonly in the treatment of acne.

5-FU—*see* Efudex.

5-FU Peeling Pulse—alternative delivery to the daily fluorouracil cream; done with weekly Jessners' Peels and a fluorouracil solution.

5-HT3 antagonists—antiemetic, which is also a selective serotonin inhibitor that inhibits the binding of serotonin to 5-HT$_3$ receptors.

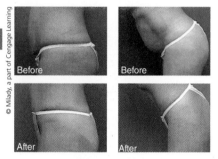

© Milady, a part of Cengage Learning

Before   Before

After   After

abdominoplasty

abdominoplasty—cosmetic surgery that removes skin and/or fat from the abdomen in order to tighten the abdomin. Also called a "tummy tuck," this surgery is typically done for women after the skin and muscles have stretched from childbirth. It is also commonly performed in both male and female patients who have had significant weight loss.

abrasive—(1) certain exfoliates; used to remove loose tissue from body surfaces (2) a substance or object that scratches or sands a rough surface.

absorbents—any product that is capable of absorbing toxins or sebum from the skin.

absorption—the uptake of one substance into another.

acanthosis (uh-can-THOH-sis)—the thickening of the stratum spinosum layer of the skin. Presents as a benign overgrowth of skin.

Accutane (isotretinoin)—trade name for oral form of vitamin A used in the treatment of acne. Often a last resort in acne care for severe instances of cystic acne.

acerola (as-uh-ROH-luh)—Barbados cherry that is high in the antioxidant vitamin C.

acetamide (uh-SET-uh-mide) **MEA**—synthetic solvent used in hair conditioners.

acetic (uh-SEE-tik) **acid**—mild organic acid, $C_2H_4O_2$, that is the main component of vinegar. Used in medicine as a styptic or astringent.

acetylcholine (uh-see-tel-KOH-leen)—a neurotransmitter and component of the parasympathetic nervous system that plays a key role in the bodys' nerve impulses. Cosmetic use of a neurotoxin inhibits the transfer of acetylcholine to the nerves controlling the muscles where it is injected, thus inhibiting the movement of the muscle.

acetylcholinesterase (uh-see-tel-koh-luh-NES-tuh-rayz)—naturally occurring enzyme that inhibits the parasympathetic nervous activity of acetylcholine.

Achard-Thiers syndrome—An uncommon disorder mainly affecting postmenopausal women, marked by diabetes mellitus and hirsutism; deep, masculine voice; facial hypertrichosis; and obesity. It is the result of excessive amounts of the male hormone androgen.

acid—substance with a low pH value; irritating. In peel solutions or AHA home solutions, a lower pH makes the product more aggressive, and a high pH makes the product milder.

acidic—any agent that has a pH less than 7.0.

acid mantle—a thin coating on the stratum corneum that is intended to protect the skin from infection. It has a pH of 4–6.5. The frequent use of products that are too alkaline or too acid changes the ability of the skin to protect itself, which can result in infection. The acid mantle is composed of sebum and sweat and is considered to be the protective barrier of the skin, protecting the body from certain types of bacteria and microorganisms.

acne conglobata (kon-GLOH-buh-tuh)—severe cystic acne that is associated with polyporpous comedones, non-inflammatory cysts, and scarring.

acné excoriée des jeunes filles (ahk-NAY ecks-core-ee-AY dayz zhewn fee)—form of acne resulting from physical manipulation of the skin, such as picking. Usually affects young girls.

acne fulminans (FUL-mee-nunz)—severe form of acne associated with confluent, inflammatory cysts and ulcers, as well as systemic symptoms.

acne mechanica—subset type of acne vulgaris brought on by friction.

acne vulgaris (vul-GAY-ris)—common inflammatory disease of the sebaceous glands and hair follicles. Acne presents with comedones, papules, pustules, and seborrhea. Scarring is

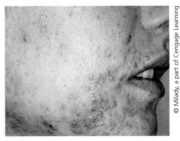

acne vulgaris

possible if there is a cystic component. Found most commonly in teenagers and young adults, yet it is not uncommon for acne vulgaris to present in adults.

Acquired Immune Deficiency Syndrome (AIDS)—the result of opportunistic infections that occur as a result of the final stages of Human Immunodeficiency Virus (HIV) and the associated compromise of the immune system.

acrochordons (ak-roh-KOR-dunz)—*see* skin tags.

A

acromegaly (ak-roh-MEG-uh-lee)—chronic condition affecting middle-aged individuals, characterized by bone enlargement of the extremities, some bones of the head and the nose, and a thickening of soft tissues of the face, including enlargement of the lips. Can be associated with changes in mood, vision (sometimes leading to blindness), and libido. Also called Marie's disease. Etiology is due to hyperfunction of the pituitary gland resulting in the overproduction of growth hormones.

actinic cheilitis (ak-TIN-ik kee-LYE-tis)—pigmentary and inflammatory condition affecting the lips; caused by repeated sun exposure.

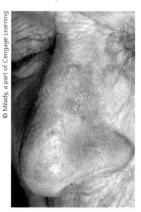

© Milady, a part of Cengage Learning

actinic keratosis

actinic keratosis (ak-TIN-ik kerr-uh-TOH-sis) **(AK)**—pink, sometimes scaly, abnormal skin lesions that are regarded to be precancerous. These lesions develop as a result of sun damage and may present on the face, ears, neck, shoulders, arms, and, most commonly, the hands.

active ingredient—skin care ingredients that cause change or action on the skin, often on the cellular level. Often these agents are defined as cosmeceuticals.

active medium—the part of a laser which absorbs and stores energy then releases it; also called impulses.

acupressure—therapeutic treatment that uses the manipulation of tissue to treat conditions that may or may not relate to the point being manipulated; for example, applying pressure to the soft tissue between the thumb and forefinger to relieve a headache.

acupuncture—therapeutic treatment that uses thin needles applied into the tissue at specific spots to treat conditions that may or may not relate to the point being manipulated. The needles are inserted at a specific location and often twisted to conduct an electric current that targets the offending condition. Acupuncture is used to treat a wide range of conditions ranging from stress to migraines.

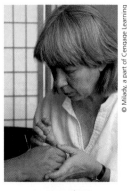

acupuncture

acute—having a rapid onset with a short but severe course.

acute coronary syndrome (ACS)—general term used for any condition that causes sudden chest pain resulting from limited blood flow to the heart.

Addison's disease—named for British physician Thomas Addison. Condition in which there exists a deficiency in the production of adrenocortical hormones by the adrenal gland. Symptoms include skin changes such as vitiligo, increased pigmentation, and black freckles on the face and neck. Other systemic symptoms include fatigue, weakness, hypotension, and gastrointestinal system disturbances such as nausea, vomiting, or diarrhea. Dehydration can occur, causing electrolyte imbalances as well as headaches, confusion, and lassitude.

adduction—the ability to move inward, as in one leg moving toward the median plane of the body.

adductor group of muscles—three powerful muscles of the upper leg that regulate adduction of the lower extremities.

adenohypophysis (ad-in-oh-hye-POF-uh-sis)—the anterior lobe of the pituitary gland.

adipose (AD-ih-pohs)—pertaining to fat.

ADR—*see* adverse drug reaction.

adrenal cortex—outer layer of the adrenal gland. This outer layer secretes specific hormones, all of which are synthesized from cholesterol. There are many hormones secreted by the cortex. These hormones are called adrenocortical hormones—more commonly known as steroids.

adrenal glands—hormone producing bodies situated above each kidney. Each gland is enclosed in a tough connective tissue

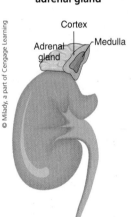

adrenal gland

adrenal medulla

called the cortex. The inside of the adrenal gland is called the medulla. It is here that the catecholamines dopamine, norepinephrine, and epinephrine are made and stored.

adrenal hyperplasia (hye-per-PLAY-zee-ah)—a group of diseases affecting the adrenal gland, resulting in the inability to produce the hormones cortisol and aldosterone.

adrenal medulla (meh-DULL-uh)—central region of the adrenal gland that stores and releases key catecholamines, including dopamine, norepinephrine, and epinephrine. The adrenal medulla is controlled by the sympathetic nervous system. These neurotransmitters are directly related to the body's stress and emotions, specifically the phenomenon "fight or flight.".

adrenocortical (uh-dree-noh-KOR-tih-kul) **insufficiency**—the suppression or lack of hormones produced in the adrenal cortex. An acute attack of adrenocortical insufficiency is also call Addisonian crisis.

adrenocorticotropic (uh-dree-noh-kor-tih-koh-TROHP-ik) **hormone (ACTH)**—hormone produced by the pituitary gland. Most associated with stress.

adrenogenital (uh-dree-noh-JEN-it-ul) **syndrome**—condition characterized by excessive androgen synthesis by the adrenal gland. Presents as precocious puberty in males, with females expressing secondary male sex characteristics such as facial hair. Can be acquired or congenital in nature.

adverse drug reaction—unintended and undesirable side effects from a drug. These effects are typically documented and well-known.

adynamic (AY-dye-nam-ik) **bone disease**—weakness or loss of bone strength. Can be caused from use of medications, a side effect of certain medical treatments, or as a symptom of an underlying disease or condition.

aerobic (ay-ROH-bik)—living or occurring only with or in the presence of oxygen.

aesculus hippocastanum—(AY-skew-lus hip-poh-CAS-tuh-num) horse chestnut; used commonly in toners and other esthetic preparations.

aesthetics—(1) the theory, philosophy, and practice of beauty (2) the study of and treatments for improving the skin and offending skin conditions.

agar (AH-gar)—originating from seaweed, a gel unaffected by bacterial enzymes; used as a culture medium, a solidifying agent, and a laxative.

aging—the universal experience of change associated with the passage of time.

aging analysis—examines how aging physically presents itself in the skin; in particular, what sorts of damaging conditions the skin has been exposed to in the past and what the results of that damage are. Aging analysis considers both intrinsic (genetic) and extrinsic (environmental) aging factors.

agonist (AG-uh-nist)—(1) the muscle that is flexed versus the muscle that is relaxed; in bending the elbow, the agonist is the bicep brachii, and the tricep is the antagonist (2) a drug that hooks onto the receptor, stimulating its function and triggering a reaction.

agoraphobia (ag-oh-roh-FOH-bee-uh)—fear of leaving the confines of one's home and interacting with others.

agranulocytes (ay-GRAN-yoo-low-sites)—a type of white blood cell, specifically a nongranular WBC.

ala (AY-luh)—a flaring, winglike cartilaginous expansion, such as on the side of each nostril or the outer ear.

alar (AY-ler)—pertaining to the nostril and associated structure, including the sphenoid bone and the sacrum.

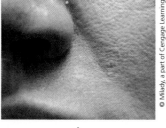

ala

© Milady, a part of Cengage Learning

albinism (AL-buh-niz-um)—A genetic, non-pathological abnormality that results in partial or complete absence of pigment in the eyes, skin, and skin's appendages, leaving skin and other tissue susceptible to solar damage.

Albumin (al-BYOO-min)—a grouping of plasma proteins, as those found in blood or egg whites. In blood, it acts to carry molecules and sustain the blood volume and blood pressure.

alchemilla (al-keh-MILL-uh) **extract**—active ingredient in medical preparations used for wound healing and anti-inflammatory purposes.

alcohol—class of organic hydrocarbons with many variations, including absolute (99%), cetyl, and grain. Used in ointments as a defatting agent; also used in beverages, medical preparations, cosmetics, and solvents.

Aldara (AL-dara)—non-antiviral, topical treatment cream or ointment for the treatment of actinic keratosis, superficial basal cell carcinoma, and HPV or warts. Operates by stimulating the body's immunologic response.

aldehyde (AL-duh-hide)—the organic byproduct that is generated when primary alcohol oxidizes. It is the intermediate step in alcohol fermentation.

aldosterone (al-doh-stih-ROHN)—mineralocorticoid hormone secreted by the adrenal cortex and responsible for metabolic regulation. Specifically, this hormone can increase the sodium absorbed by the kidneys, which in turn affects the levels of potassium, chloride, and bicarbonate. The increase of sodium also affects blood pressure and blood volume.

algae extract—considered an active ingredient in skin care preparations; said to improve moisture in the epidermis. Derived from algae.

alimentary (al-uh-MEN-tuh-ree) **canal**—the intestinal tract.

alkaline—anything that has a pH greater than 7.0.

alkalinity—pertaining to an agent with alkaline properties; the degree to which an agent's pH is greater than 7.0.

alkaloids—organic, nitrogen-based plant substances used in medical and esthetic preparations.

alkyloamides (AL-kih-loh-am-ides)—an ingredient used for thickening; commonly in shampoos and liquid hand and body cleansers.

allantoin (uh-LAN-toh-in)—humectant and anti-irritant derived from comfrey root. Can also be produced synthetically through the oxidation of uric acid. Used to promote wound healing.

allergenic extract—protein-based substance that creates an allergic response.

aloe barbadensis (bar-buh-DEN-sis)—also called aloe vera; non-irritating plant-based gel derived from many species of the aloe plant. May have healing and soothing properties.

alopecia (al-oh-PEE-shee-uh)—disease that presents as partial or total hair loss. May be a symptom of a disease, an independent condition, or a side effect of medication or chemotherapy.

alpha-glucosidase (gloo-KOH-sih-days) **inhibitors**—group of medications used to treat diabetes by slowing the breakdown of sugars in the body.

alpha hydroxy (hye-DROK-see) **acids (AHA)**—mild organic acids used in cosmeceutical products and as peeling agents. AHAs "unglue" cells in the epidermis, allowing keratinocytes to be shed at the stratum granulosum, providing skin with a healthier texture.

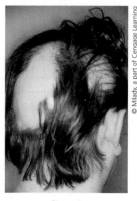

alopecia

aluminium oxide—type of crystal used in microdermabrasion machines.

aluminosilicates—minerals, specifically aluminum and silicone, found in clay.

Alzheimer's (ALTZ-hye-merz) **disease**—named for German neurologist Alois Alzheimer. A chronic, progressive neurological condition characterized by the onset of dementia at age 65 or older. Presenile form usually begins between 40 and 60 years of age.

ambergris (AM-ber-gris)—substance cast off by sperm whales, used in the production of perfume.

American National Standard Institute (ANSI)—a voluntary organization of experts that establishes industry consensus standards in various fields, particularly with regard to the use of lasers and lights in plastic surgery or dermatology.

amino acid—protein building unit that helps break down simple sugars and fats; contains both an amino group and a carboxylic group. There are 20 amino acids necessary for human life. There are essential amino acids and nonessential amino acids. Essential amino acids are supplied by food; nonessential amino acids are created within the body.

aminolevulinic acid—polypeptide that is thought to be the source of certain brain cancers.

A

ammonium laureth sulphate—a surfactant in shampoos, cleansers, and body washes.

ammonium lauryl sulphate—a surfactant; more irritating than ammonium laureth sulphate.

ammonium pareth–25 sulphate—a surfactant used for foaming and cleansing.

ampere (AM-peer)—basic unit of electric current that measures the current's force.

ampholyte (AM-foh-light)—any substance that can chemically react as both a base and an acid depending on the pH of the solution it interacts with.

amphoteric (am-foh-TER-ik)—pertaining to an ampholyte.

anabolic-androgenic steroids (AAS)—steroids that promote muscle growth with the aid of hormones, particularly testosterone, and increase protein synthesis; used to illicitly enhance athletic performance.

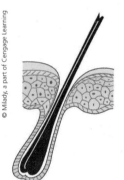
anagen phase

anabolism (uh-NAB-uh-lizm)—productive phase of metabolism; the opposite of catabolism.

anaerobic (an-ay-ROH-bik)—not requiring oxygen to exist.

anagen phase—the phase of hair growth in which growth is actually occurring.

analgesic (an-ul-JEE-zik)—a pain reliever; both narcotic and non-narcotic pain-relieving drugs.

ananas sativus (uh-NAN-us sah-TYE-vus)—pineapple extract; acidic nature assists with exfoliation of the skin in many cosmetic preparations.

anaphoresis (an-uh-foh-REE-sis)—(1) the movement of particles toward the positive pole (2) a reduction in the activity of sweat glands.

anaphylactic (an-uh-fih-LAK-tik) **reactions**—*see* anaphylaxis.

anaphylaxis (an-uh-fih-LAK-sis)—serious hypersensitive allergic reaction characterized by respiratory distress, hypotension, edema, rash, tachycardia, and possible death. Immediate medical attention is necessary.

anastomose (uh-NAS-tuh-mohz)—joining of parts end to end, whether natural or surgical; the connection point of different parts of a branching network.

anatomy—the study of the body structure.

A

ancillary material—in the case of cosmetics, a substance such as a filler, additive, or carrier that is not the primary active ingredient.

androgenic—causing or referring to masculine features, as in male secondary sex characteristics such as facial hair growth.

androgens (AN-droh-jenz)—hormones that promote the production of male secondary sex characteristics.

anemia—state characterized by a decrease in the number of red blood cells. It is a symptom of disease processes but not a disease itself. Diseases that present with anemia include hemorrhage, hemolytic diseases, hypersplenism, loss of bone marrow, or bone marrow failures from the decrease in red blood cell production through a disease process.

anesthesia—the administration of a medication intended to cause temporary loss of sensation with or without loss of consciousness. Can be administered through topical, inhalation, and intravenous delivery methods.

anesthetic—any substance that causes a temporary loss of sensation with or without loss of consciousness.

angina (an-JYE-nuh)—chest pain resulting from lack of oxygen supplied to the heart. Typically, the sensation starts around the heart and radiates up the individual's left chest and down the left arm. Left untreated, it can be grave.

angioedema (an-jee-oh-eh-DEE-mah)—allergic condition characterized by hives and swelling of the skin. Typically benign and associated with foods, drugs, stings, molds, or the skin's reaction to changes in the environment such as cold, pressure, or exercise.

anion (AN-eye-un)—negatively charged particle or ion; the opposite of cation.

ankylosing spondylitis (an-kih-LOH-sing spon-dih-LYE-tis)—chronic condition characterized by stiffening, inflammation, and, in extreme cases, fusion of the vertebrae in the spine resulting in loss of movement.

annular—ring-shaped; used to define ligaments.

anorexia—condition characterized by weight loss stemming from a loss of appetite or refusal to eat. Anorexia is also seen in many diseases such as depression, fevers, disorders of the gastrointestinal tract, alcoholism, and drug addiction.

antacid—any agent that neutralizes stomach acid.

antagonist—a muscle or muscle group that counteracts the motions of another muscle group; opposite of synergist.

anterior—situated before or in front of something else.

anthelmintic (an-thel-MIN-tik)—an herb or agent that destroys and dispels worms, parasites, fungus, and yeast from the intestines.

anthranilates (an-THRAN-il-ayts)—weak UVB filters. They absorb mainly in the near UVA portion of the light spectrum.

antianginals—class of drugs that are used to prevent the onset of an angina-related chest pain. Most commonly amyl nitrate or nitroglycerine; *see* angina.

antianxiety drugs—any drug that prevents or limits the severity of the symptoms of anxiety or an anxiety disorder.

antiasthmatics—any drug that prevents or limits the severity of the symptoms of an asthma attack.

antibacterial—inhibiting the increase and duplication of bacteria.

antibilious—any agent that fights nausea and discomfort caused by an oversecretion of bile.

antibiotic—a natural or synthetic substance that is toxic to or inhibiting to microbial organisms; used to fight infection.

antibody—primary immunologic response in which glycoproteins are secreted into the blood or lymph in response to an antigenic stimulus, such as a bacterium, virus, parasite, or transplanted organ, in order to neutralize the antigen.

anticholinergics (an-tye-koh-luh-NUR-jiks)—agents that block parasympathetic nerve impulses. These drugs may act to limit spasms and cramping of the digestive or urinary tract, for example.

anticonvulsants—any drug that prevents or limits the severity of convulsive activity resulting from certain neurological conditions.

antidepressants—any drug that prevents or limits the severity of the symptoms of depression.

antidiarrheal—any agent that remedies diarrhea.

antielastase (an-tye-ih-LAS-tayz)—slows down the action of elastase.

antiemetics (an-tye-ee-MET-ik)—any drug that prevents or limits the severity of the symptoms of nausea and vomiting.

antigen—a protein marker on the cell that defines the type (skin, liver, kidney). These markers stimulate production of antibodies when detected. Primary immunologic response that recognizes the invasion of foreign bodies.

antigen agglutination (uh-gloot-in-AY-shun AN-tih-jen)—antibody reaction in which an antigen sticks together with a perceived offending antibody. Most often occurs when the wrong blood type is transfused, causing the cells to clump together and making the blood transfusion unviable.

antihelix—the inside curve of the outer ear cartilage.

antihistamines—any drug that blocks the action of histamine, a naturally occurring amino acid. Use particularly in allergic responses.

antilithic—any agent or substance that helps to prevent calcium stones in the kidney and bladder.

antimetabolite—a class of drugs most often used to treat rapidly growing tumors, but can also be used to treat otherwise uncontrollable skin eruptions.

antimicrobials—any substance that has the ability to prevent or kill microorganisms.

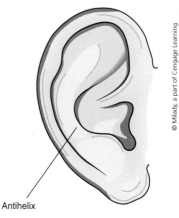

Antihelix

© Milady, a part of Cengage Learning

A

antioxidant facials—skin treatment that focuses on the symptoms of the prematurely aged skin using antioxidant products including vitamin C, vitamin E, hyaluronic acid, or other nourishing ingredients.

antioxidants—vitamins and substances that neutralize free radical oxidation or deterioration; for example, vitamins A, C, and E.

antiperspirants—herbs or chemicals that hamper perspiration.

antipsychotic—any drug that prevents or limits the severity of the symptoms of psychosis.

antipyretic (an-tih-pye-RET-ik)—drug that reduces fever.

antirheumatic—agents that may relieve rheumatism, a general term for any condition characterized by chronic and acute pain and inflammation of the joint and surrounding muscles.

antiseptic—a substance or agent used to decontaminate surfaces, objects, and wounds; inhibits the growth of bacteria.

antispasmodics—*see* anticonvulsants.

antitoxin—used in response to biologic toxins.

antiulcer drugs—any drug that prevents or limits the severity of the symptoms of peptic ulcers.

aorta (ay-OR-tuh)—primary and largest artery that carries blood from the heart to the auxiliary arteries of the trunk and limbs as well as the body at large.

aortic (ay-OR-tik) **semilunar valve**—made of three cusps, it prevents blood from flowing back into the heart (*see* Figure 2.17 on page 29).

aphthous stomatitis (AF-thus stoh-muh-TYE-tis)—recurrent ulcers of the oral cavity; also known as a "canker sore."

apnea—temporary ceasing of normal breathing function resulting in the intake of carbon dioxide and diminished oxygen levels; often happens while sleeping.

apocrine (AP-uh-krin) **sweat glands**—larger of the sweat glands, which are housed in auxillary (under the arm), pubic, and perianal areas. These sweat glands open into hair follicles rather than onto the skin.

aponeurosis (ap-uh-noo-ROH-sis)—thick, flat, and tendon-like deep tissues that attach bones to muscles.

apoptosis (ah-pup-TOH-sis)—cell death caused by injury, disease, heat, or normal pre-programmed cell death.

appendages—any anatomical structures associated with a larger structure; for the skin, its appendages include nails, hair, and sebaceous and sweat glands.

appendicular skeleton—the bones of the limbs.

applied cosmetics—cosmetics that are easily put on and removed; opposite of permanent makeup.

arachidonic (ayr-eh-kih-DON-ik) **acid**—an essential fatty acid; also known as Omega–6.

arachis (AYR-eh-kis) **oil**—peanut oil; a carrier product for skin care products and some topical medical preparations.

arbutin (ar-BYOO-ten)—A glycoside found in the bearberry and related plants; bleaching agent for the skin; tyrosine inhibitor. Found in cosmetic preparations.

arciform (AR-suh-form)—shaped like a partial circle.

argon—a chemical element in the form of an inert gas used in the creation of early lasers.

arnica—popular botanical used orally and topically for anti-inflammatory and anticoagulant purposes; also used as an antiseptic, astringent, and antimicrobial.

aromatherapy—the practice of using essential oils from natural botanicals in lotions, inhalants, and serums in an effort to affect mood and promote health of mind and body.

aromatic—to have an aroma, whether or not it be pleasing to the senses.

arrector pili (PYE-lye) **muscle**—involuntary muscle of the skin that attaches to the hair follicle. The arrector pili muscle contracts when the body is cold, creating "goosebumps."

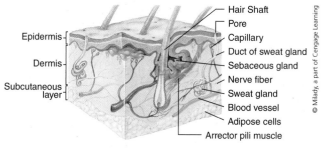

Epidermis — Hair Shaft — Pore — Capillary — Duct of sweat gland — Sebaceous gland — Nerve fiber — Sweat gland — Blood vessel — Adipose cells — Arrector pili muscle

Dermis

Subcutaneous layer

© Milady, a part of Cengage Learning

arrector pili

arrhythmia—abnormal heartbeat.

artefactual dermatoses—condition characterized by self-inflicted skin injuries.

arteries—network of blood vessels that transport oxygenated blood to tissues, organs, and cells (*see* illustration on next page).

arterioles—smallest component of the blood vessel network, which connects with capillary beds (*see* illustration on next page).

arteriovenous communications—communication which occurs between the arteries and the veins; intended to regulate the flow of oxygenated and deoxygenated blood to the heart and throughout the body (*see* illustration on page 109).

arthralgia (ar-THRAL-jee-uh)—joint pain.

atrioventricular valves—valves that prevent blood flow from the atria back into the ventricles of the heart (*see* Figure 2.17 on page 29).

ascomycetes (as-kuh-MY-seets)—true fungi; yeast and molds.

ascorbic (uh-SKOR-bik) **acid**—*see* Vitamin C.

ascorbyl palmitate (as-KOR-bil PAL-mih-tayt)—fat-soluble form of ascorbic acid.

asepsis (uh-SEP-sis)—sterile; disease-producing organisms are not present; state of being free from pathogens.

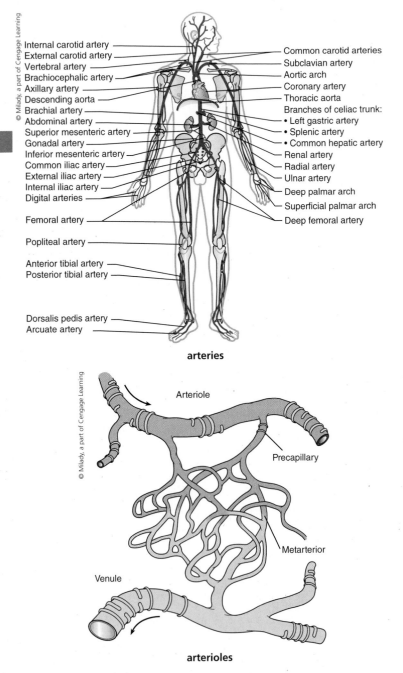

Internal carotid artery
External carotid artery
Vertebral artery
Brachiocephalic artery
Axillary artery
Descending aorta
Brachial artery
Abdominal artery
Superior mesenteric artery
Gonadal artery
Inferior mesenteric artery
Common iliac artery
External iliac artery
Internal iliac artery
Digital arteries

Femoral artery

Popliteal artery

Anterior tibial artery
Posterior tibial artery

Dorsalis pedis artery
Arcuate artery

Common carotid arteries
Subclavian artery
Aortic arch
Coronary artery
Thoracic aorta
Branches of celiac trunk:
• Left gastric artery
• Splenic artery
• Common hepatic artery
Renal artery
Radial artery
Ulnar artery
Deep palmar arch
Superficial palmar arch
Deep femoral artery

arteries

Arteriole

Precapillary

Metarterior

Venule

arterioles

© Milady, a part of Cengage Learning

A

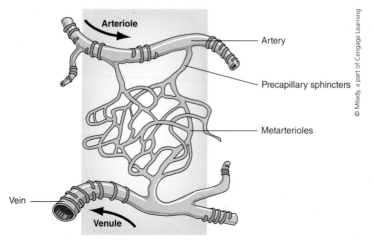

arteriovenous communications

ASPS (American Society of Plastic Surgeons)—organization of plastic surgeons that defines ethical codes and keeps statistical data for the industry.

asthenia—weakness or lack of strength.

asthma—a chronic condition in which airway constriction results from a triggering event. Triggering events can include drugs, exercise and inhaling or consuming allergens.

astringent—product used to restore the natural acidity of the skin. It accomplishes as much by protein coagulation. Most astringents are salts of metals.

asymptomatic—presenting without symptoms.

ataxia—defective muscle coordination.

athlete's foot—contagious fungal infection of the feet; also called tinea pedis.

atopic—displaced or out of place; malpositioned.

atopic dermatitis—a skin irritation or rash of unknown etiology; also called eczema. Presents as macules or coalescing plaques and itching. Can be exacerbated by scratching and other physical manipulation.

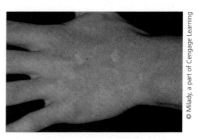

atopic dermatitis

atrial flutter—cardiac arrhythmia characterized

by a rapid (usually 300 beats per minute) activity of the atrial muscles.

atrioventricular conduction—component of the cardiac electrical system during which there is forward conduction from the axia-ventricles.

atrium—one of the two upper chambers of the heart that receive blood (plural atria).

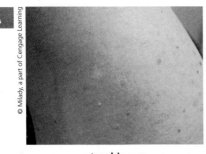

atrophic scar

atrophic scar—flat, small, round, and generally inverted scars. Usually seen in acne or chickenpox scarring.

atrophy—a decrease in size due to lack of use; loss of muscle tissue and tone, most often from inactivity, blood supply, or disease.

atypical—unusual or dysfunctional.

autoclave—machine that provides moist heat ster-ilization.

autoimmune disease—general name for any condition that occurs when the body becomes intolerant of its own antigen markers or when the immune system fails to recognize itself.

autologous—derived or harvested from the same species in which it is implanted; for example, human collagen is implanted into humans to remove wrinkles and lines from the skin.

autonomic nervous system—part of the peripheral nervous system that helps to control involuntary movement, such as that of the heart.

autotrophs—organisms that are self-nourishing. Grow with the absence of organic compounds. Pertinent to green plants or bacteria.

avascular—lacking blood vessels; synonomous with the stratum corneum.

avobenzone (BMDM—butyl methoxydibenzoylmethane)—chemical sunscreen agent; works by absorbing UVA rays.

axial skeleton—bones of the skull, vertebrae, and thorax.

axillae (ak-SIL-ee)—underarm.

A

axillary incision—when the incision is made in the underarm area, as when done for breast augmentation surgery.

ayurveda (eye-er-VAY-duh)—Indian theory and system of traditional medicine dating back to 2500 B.C.; known as the science of living.

azelaic (AH-zuh-lay-ik) **acid**—an antibacterial agent, comedolytic, and anti-inflammatory agent that is usually used for acne treatment. It also has shown promise in minimizing dyschromia. Derived from wheat, rye, and barley.

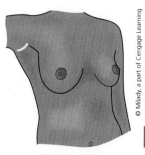

axillary incision

© Milady, a part of Cengage Learning

A

azulene (AH-zoo-leen)—a distilled oil and naturally occurring blue pigment; part of the chamomile essential oil. Known for its fragrance and blue color, azulene oils have long been used in aromatherapy, chromatherapy, and cosmetic preparations.

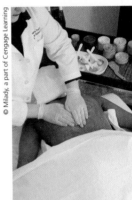

back facials

back facials—treatments that involve cleansing, toning, exfoliating, masking, extraction, and massaging the back side of the body; similar to a standard facial and involving the same steps as well as the same products.

bacteria—single-celled organisms that are flexible and reproduce and mature quickly. They are also some of the oldest known species on the planet. Some bacteria are responsible for disease whereas others are relatively harmless.

bactericide—destroys bacteria but not its spores.

bacteriostatic—slows the growth of bacterial organisms.

bacterium—*see* bacteria.

Baker-Gordon solution—deep phenol peel solution for high degrees of photodamage. It is a technique-sensitive treatment that has great potential for risk for scarring to the client.

balneotherapy—therapeutic water treatment that involves soaking with seawater, freshwater, or thermal springs.

balsam—tree resin used for healing and soothing.

barbiturates—highly addictive central nervous system depressants.

bariatric (bayr-ee-AH-trik) **surgery**—weight loss surgery commonly referred to as gastric bypass; a process whereby drastic weight loss is accomplished.

barrier creams—creams meant to protect the skin from the dangers posed by the external environment.

basal cell carcinoma (BCC)—a slow-growing tumor that generally does not metastasize. It is the most common form of skin cancer, which usually occurs in regions of repeated sunburn. Begins as a shiny area that may appear as a clogged pore. Sometimes it will have a central depression. In other cases it presents as a skin ulcer that bleeds.

basal layer—*see* stratum basale.

basal zone—living layer of dividing cells that continuously change and push upward.

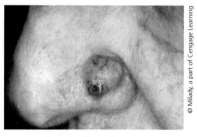

basal cell carcinoma

B

basophils (BAY-soh-fils)—granulated white blood cell.

bayberry—botanical that is considered antibacterial, used primarily in therapeutic acne treatments.

bearberry—botanical used in skin care products and peeling agents to treat dyschromias.

bearberry extract—has been used for antiseptic and anti-inflammatory purposes. Also useful for skin eruptions such as acne.

benign—not recurrent, progressive, or malicious to one's health; not cancerous.

bentonite—non-toxic clay used in masks and gels.

benzodiazepines (ben-zoh-dye-AZ-uh-peens)—group of drugs with a sedative effect; predominantly used to treat anxiety and sleep disorders.

benzoic (ben-ZOH-ik) **acid**—a preservative especially effective against molds and yeast.

benzoin (BEN-zoh-in)—balsamic resin from trees; essential oil; antibacterial, anti-irritant, antipruritic.

benzophenone (ben-zoh-fih-NOHN)—chemical absorbers that respond to UV light by generating a free radical capable of rapid polymerization. Agent commonly used in sunscreens.

benzoyl peroxide—bactericidal and keratolytic agent used in home treatment of low grade acne. It is used in concentrations of 2.5%, 5%, and 10% in many over-the-counter acne treatments. It may cause redness and irritation in some clients.

benzyl alcohol—a preservative effective against bacteria.

beta-carotene—from carrot oil; it has antioxidant, pigment, and photo protection properties.

beta-hydroxy acid (BHA)—isometrically distinct relative of alpha hydroxyl acids; in other words, they are separated by only one carbon atom. Used in the care of acne.

betaines (BEE-tuh-eens)—surfactant; builds viscosity in products; causes foaming. Mostly used in soaps and shampoos.

beta-peel—20% or 30% salicylic acid peel solution.

BHA—*see* beta-hydroxy acid.

bicarbonate solution—Any salt containing HCO_3 anion; an example is carbonic acid, an acid created from the mixture of water and carbon dioxide.

bicep brachialis (bray-kee-AL-is)—muscle of the upper arm which is responsible for flexing the arm and rotating the arm.

bicuspid valve—heart valve located between the left atrium and left ventricle and regulates backflow between the two chambers. Also called the mitral valve. (*See* Figure 2.17 on page 29).

biliopancreatic (bil-ee-oh-pan-kree-AT-ik) **diversion**—process by which the stomach size is reduced during bariatric surgery.

binocular—relating to both eyes, as in "binocular vision."

biochemistry—the chemical study of living plants, animals, and humans.

biocide—any substance or agent that kills organisms without prejudice.

biodegradation—a biological action that breaks down materials.

biohazard—processing risk or danger to humans, plants, or animals.

biologic—pertaining to the study of living beings, plants, or animals.

biopsy—a section of tissue taken for examination. Most often, the tissue is obtained with a needle, though surgical ex-

— Biceps brachialis

© Milady, a part of Cengage Learning

B

traction is also used. The purpose of doing so is to obtain a diagnosis.

bipolar disorder—mental condition characterized by periods of high activity and then severe depression; previously known as manic-depressive syndrome.

black box warning—Also known as a "black label warning" or "boxed warning." It is a warning that accompanies certain drugs if the FDA feels that the drug can cause serious side effects or life-threatening events. It is called "black box" due to the thick black line that surrounds the warning information. It is the strongest warning the FDA can issue.

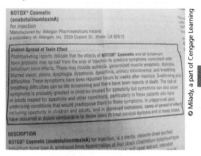

black box warning

blackberry extract—used as an astringent in esthetic preparations, especially for acne care.

black label warning—*see* black box warning.

blanch—rapid loss of coloration.

blanket wraps—the application of a covering after a body treatment in the spa to maintain heat or to cool the body to aid in the penetration of active ingredients.

blastocyst (BLAS-tuh-sist)—stage in early embryonic development during which implantation of the embryo into the lining of the uterus occurs.

blending—hair removal technique that transitions wanted into unwanted hair, preventing a severe transition.

blepharospasm (BLEF-or-uh-spaz-um)— abnormal spastic movement; for example, blinking or twitching of the orbicularis oculis. Usually a result of frequent and prolonged eye strain.

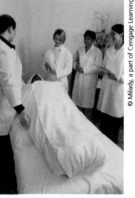

blanket wraps

Bloodborne Pathogen Act—law that hospitals and medical employers must follow when taking care of patients. It was enacted to reduce the transmission of Hepatitis B and other bloodborne pathogens and to provide for the safety of employees who may come in contact with medical waste.

blood-borne pathogens—infectious microorganisms that can be transmitted to others through direct contact with blood or body fluids. Examples of blood-borne pathogens include HIV and Hepatitis C.

blood-brain barrier (BBB)—mechanism that alters the permeability of brain capillaries so that some substances, such as certain drugs, are prevented from entering brain tissue, whereas other substances, such as oxygen, are allowed to enter freely.

bloodletting—archaic and irrelevant medical treatment that released blood from the body as a means of treating disease.

blood lipids—concentration of fat in the blood.

blood plasma—liquid component of blood in which only platelet cells (needed for clotting factors) remain; it is a clear, dense, straw-colored fluid.

blood platelets—a component of blood, essential for clotting.

blood pressure—measurable force exerted by the blood on arterial vessel walls related to the degree to which the heart pumps the blood through the body. Individuals can have variable levels of blood pressure. It can be high following periods of activity or low during sleep. Furthermore, different individuals may have varying blood pressure at rest. High or low resting blood pressure may be indicative of a number of conditions or diseases.

body dysmorphic disorder (BDD)—chronic mental health disorder that causes individuals to be inappropriately preoccupied with their appearance. Those affected with BDD are contraindicated for most esthetic procedures.

body-focused repetitive disorder (BFRD)—disorder

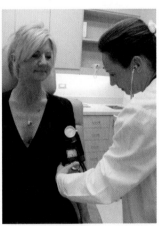

© Milady, a part of Cengage Learning

blood pressure

characterized by repeated manipulation of a body part because of a perceived flaw; for example, picking or cutting.

body masque (mask)—therapeutic body treatment in which exfoliating, hydrating detoxification agent(s) is/are applied to the entire body, much the way it would be applied to the face. Often, similar product and techniques are used.

body sculpting—generic term for the collective surgeries used to reduce excess skin and fat in patients who have undergone massive weight loss. Can also be used to describe the process of liposuction or liposculpting.

botanical—pertaining to herbs or organic agents derived from plants.

Botox (botulism toxin or clostridium botulium)—trade name for botulism toxin that is injected into the wrinkle-causing muscles. The toxin blocks the release of acetylcholine, which would otherwise signal the muscle to contract, thus paralyzing the injected muscle, in turn neutralizing the wrinkle. Botox is FDA approved for the treatment of glabella frown lines but is also used for the treatment of crow's feet, horizontal forehead lines, and upper and lower lip lines.

botulinum (boch-uh-LYE-num) **toxin type A**—see Botox or Dysport.

bovine—derived from cows.

bovine collagen—heterologous collagen that is derived from the hide of cows.

brachioplasty—plastic surgery of the arms by which excess skin is

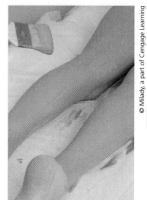

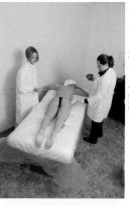

body masque

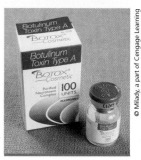

Botox

B

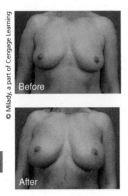

breast augmentation

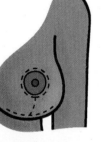

breast lifts

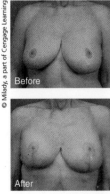

breast reduction

removed; often resulting in significant scarring.

branding—a trademark or an attempt to associate a product with a company that produces a product that other companies produce as well; for example, Kleenex.

breast augmentation—type of cosmetic surgery whereby a silicone or saline implant is placed behind the breast to enhance the overall size, shape, or contour of the breast.

breast lifts—type of cosmetic surgery by which sagging or drooping breasts are brought up higher on the chest, resulting in a more youthful appearance.

breast reduction—type of cosmetic surgery involving removal of breast tissue to reduce the size.

bridge—narrow band of cartilage, link of the junction of the nasal bones.

broad spectrum—a wide range, usually in reference to medications and their scope of treatment or efficacy.

bronchodilators—group of drugs that are used to reverse acute bronchial constriction by dilating the bronchi, thus allowing freer air flow.

bronchogenic cancers—subset of lung cancer that originates in the bronchus.

browlift—type of cosmetic surgery that raises the area from the eyebrows to the hairline, thus reducing the appearance of lines on the forehead and a drooping brow.

btu (British thermal unit)—unit of measure for heat energy.

buffers—any agents that offset the strength or performance of another chemical or substance; examples are neutralizers on peels or hydrogen ions added to solutions to change their pH.

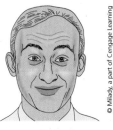

candidate for browlift

B

bulge region—above the papilla that produces follicular stem cells and is responsible for the growth and development of the hair follicle.

bulking agents—products used to extend volume; clays, calcium carbonate, talc.

bulla (BUL-uh)—skin eruption that presents as a large fluid-filled blister greater than 1 cm.

burn—skin injury that occurs as a result of intense thermal, electrical, or acidic agents. Burns are typically classified according to how far they penetrate the skin: first degree (superficial), second degree (partial thickness), and third degree (full thickness).

Burow's soaks—solution of aluminum acetate–soaked cloths applied to weeping wounds with the intent of drying them out.

butylated hydroxyanisole (BYOO-til-ayt-ed hye-drok-see-AN-uh-sohl)—preservative and antioxidant. Not to be confused with beta hydroxy acid.

butyrospermum parkii (BYOO-too-roh-sperm-um PAR-kye)—also known as shea butter; commonly used as a moisturizer in cosmetic preparations.

C—Celsius; unit of temperature measurement.

calamine—mild agent used to relive itching; mild astringent with cooling qualities.

calcium—metallic element that is silver and white in color; symbol Ca. Carried through the blood in the body and works in conjunction with vitamin D to enable bone growth.

calcium carbonate—chalk; naturally occurring in limestone, but also in coral and marble. Used as an abrasive in toothpastes and other personal products.

calcium hydroxylapatite (hye-drok-zihl-AP-uh-tite)—naturally occurring mineral that is found mostly in bones.

calendula (kuh-LEN-juh-luh) **extract (officinali)**—herb used to treat irritated or inflamed skin. It has anti-inflammatory and antiseptic properties; also called marigold extract.

calibration—to determine the accuracy of a machine or instrument by comparing certain information to a known standard. For example, when discussing laser equipment, this means to ensure a machine's accuracy; to calibrate.

calorie—unit of heat measurement.

camphor (cinnamomum camphora)—used as anesthetic, antiseptic, and anti-inflammatory agent. Also useful as a toner with astringent and cooling properties.

cancer—malignant neoplasm that occurs in over 200 different types. Marked by uncontrolled growth and spreading of the abnormal cells that invade nearby organs and tissues. Proliferation of abnormal cell growth associated with cancer may be caused by a variety of factors including genetics, viruses, radiation, ultraviolet light, and exposure to certain toxic chemicals. Diagnosis of cancer is made in a variety of ways, most often through biopsy or devices, such as ultrasound, meant to see through hollow organs. Treatment is often complex and complicated, but often involves targeted radiation and/or chemotherapy. Prognosis is variant and often depends where the cancer is, if it has metastasized, and how advanced it has become.

candelilla (kan-duhl-EE-uh) **wax**—vegetable wax derived from the candelilla plant. Commonly used in waxing treatments.

candidiasis (kan-dih-DYE-uh-sis)—a skin infection characterized by presence of yeast-like fungi that reproduce by means of budding.

cannula (KAN-yuh-luh)—a tube that allows the removal or delivery of a substance or fluid. For example, in plastic surgery a liposuction cannula is used to remove fat. Oxygen is delivered to patients through a cannula as well.

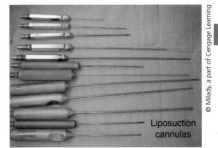

Liposuction cannulas

© Milady, a part of Cengage Learning

cannula

capillaries—tiny blood vessels that connect arterioles and venules and where gases, nutrients, and other substances are exchanged.

capsicum—herb used for circulatory and digestive system; also called Spanish pepper.

capsid—the outer protein cover around the central core of a virus that encapsulates the genetic material of a virus and helps the virus to attack susceptible cells.

capsular contracture—scar tissue that forms around a breast implant, resulting in a hardening of the breast tissue.

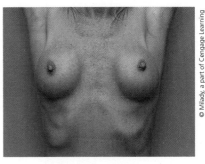

© Milady, a part of Cengage Learning

capsular contracture

carrageenan (kar-uh-GEE-nun)—edible seaweed.

carbohydrates—a macronutrient required by the body. Group of substances including sugars, glycogen, starches, dextrins and celluloses. They function as the body's primary source of fuel and can be found in every tissue in the body, but primarily in the liver and muscles, where they can be dispatched as reserve energy when necessary. Carbohydrates contain only carbon, oxygen, and hydrogen. Common in fruits, grains, and nuts, carbohydrates are thought to be the most common chemical compounds on earth.

carbolic acid—*see* phenol.

carbomer-934—a crosslinked polymer used as a thickener in moisturizers, creams, and other esthetic products.

carbocisteine (kar-boh-SIS-teen)—mucolytic that reduces the viscosity of mucous. Used in the treatment of bronchitis, asthma, and COPD.

carotenoids (kuh-ROT-in-oyds)—naturally occurring organic pigments.

carboxymethyl cellulose—a thickener for bath products and creams.

carbuncle—inflamed, painful, pus-filled skin eruptions with systemic symptoms including fevers and increased white blood cells. Known to originate from opportunistic Staphylococci infection and treatable with broad-range antibiotics.

carcinogen—any substance that causes cancer.

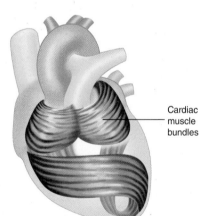

© Milady, a part of Cengage Learning

Cardiac muscle bundles

cardiac fibers—flexible cells that make up cardiac muscles; found exclusively in the heart.

cardiac muscles—tissue type found exclusively in the heart and a key agent in the ability of the heart to perform, as it allows the heart to expand and contract.

cardiovascular system—the entirety of the heart and all the blood vessels. (*see* illustration on next page)

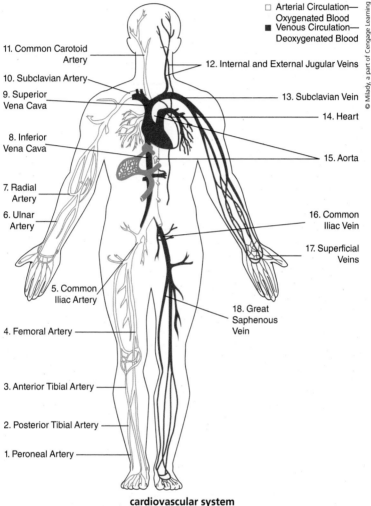

□ Arterial Circulation—
  Oxygenated Blood
■ Venous Circulation—
  Deoxygenated Blood

© Milady, a part of Cengage Learning

11. Common Carotoid Artery

10. Subclavian Artery

9. Superior Vena Cava

8. Inferior Vena Cava

7. Radial Artery

6. Ulnar Artery

5. Common Iliac Artery

4. Femoral Artery

3. Anterior Tibial Artery

2. Posterior Tibial Artery

1. Peroneal Artery

12. Internal and External Jugular Veins

13. Subclavian Vein

14. Heart

15. Aorta

16. Common Iliac Vein

17. Superficial Veins

18. Great Saphenous Vein

cardiovascular system

carminative (kar-MIN-uh-tiv)—any agent that relieves intestinal gas; for example, chamomile or peppermint.

carmine—from the female Coccu cacti insect; used for red dye in cosmetic formulations.

carnauba (kar-NOO-buh) **wax**—the hardest and most widely used vegetable wax; derived from the leaves of the carnauba palm tree.

carotene—used for a red-orange coloring, found in nature, but used in cosmetic formulations.

carrier—(1) has a specific pathogenic organism or mutated gene (2) the substance that a topical product may float in (3) an individual who harbors a disease.

cartilage—hard connective tissue considered to be part of the skeletal system.

casein (KAY-seen)—milk protein; when coagulated it becomes cheese. Also used as an emulsifier in cosmetic preparations.

catagen phase—the transition stage of the hair's growth cycle; the period between the growth and resting phases.

catalyst—an agent or substance that initiates or accelerates a chemical reaction with itself being compromised.

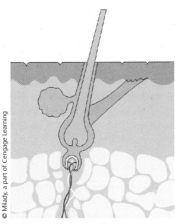

© Milady, a part of Cengage Learning

catagen phase

cataphoresis (kat-uh-fuh-REE-sis)—transmission of ions through the skin with an electrical current.

catechol-0-methyltransferase inhibitors (KAT-ih-kol zero METH-uhl TRANS-fuh-rays)—an agent that breaks down levodopa, allowing greater availability in the central nervous system. Used in the treatment of Parkinson's disease.

cathartic—(1) to move (2) agent that facilitates evacuation of the bowel.

cathode pole—device used to negatively charge ions.

cation—positively charged particle.

caustic—**soda** *see* sodium hydroxide.

cautery—instrument used for abnormal tissue destruction with use of heat or electricity.

cell—the basic unit of life; protoplasm with a nucleus or nuclear material. Cells make up all the tissues and structures in living beings. They originate from other cells through cell division and are specialized to perform certain and unique functions.

cell differentiation—cells that are developed within the body for different reasons; *see* stem cells.

cellophane body wrap—a body treatment that uses a thin plastic material to assist in active ingredient penetration through the principle of occlusion.

cellulitis—a spreading inflammation of cells or cellular material within connective tissue. Typically begins as a small infection of the skin and progresses to systemic symptoms such as fever. As the inflammation moves through the tissues, the process is then defined as cellulitis. Those at risk include the elderly and those with a compromised immune system.

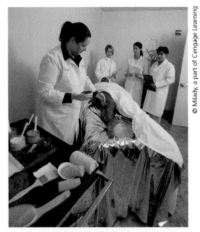

cellophane body wrap

cellulose gum—a thickening and stabilizing product.

Center for Device and Radiologic Health (CDRH)—a regulatory agency within the FDA that has specific responsibility for standardizing the design, research, manufacturing, and distribution of radiation emitting medical devices.

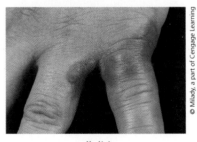

cellulitis

Centers for Disease Control and Prevention (CDC)—a government agency that conducts research on disease and implements protocols and policies to ensure public safety.

central nervous system stimulants—any drug that increases nervous system activity.

centrofacial—in the center of the face.

centrifuge—a machine used to spin liquids or blood into two separate solutions; solids (blood cells) and liquids (plasma).

ceramides (seh-RAM-ides)—a class of lipids that does not contain glycerol; found in cosmetics and assist in the reduction of transepidermal water loss or TEWL.

cervical dystonia—prolonged, repetitive muscle contractions that may cause twisting or jerking movements of the neck.

ceteareth (Sa-tear-reth)—an emollient, emulsifier, and lubricant for skin care products.

cetearyl alcohol—an emulsifying wax from plant or natural waxes; used as an emollient.

cetearyl glucoside—emulsifying substance from corn and coconut.

cetrimonium (set-trih-MOH-nee-uhm) **chloride**—surfactant used in conditioners; may also be an antiseptic or preservative.

chalazion (kah-LAY-zee-on)—a cyst in the eyelid.

chamomile—herb that is known to be effective as a bactericidal, anti-inflammatory, anti-itching, and antiseptic agent. There are many different types of chamomile plants, including German chamomile and Roman chamomile.

chelating agents—*see* chelatory agent.

chelatory agent—a substance that binds minerals to itself. In cosmetic manufacturing, it refers to chemicals that mop up free ions, such as metals, in formulae and inhibit them from causing deterioration of the product; also called a chelating agent.

chemical peeling—the controlled use of chemicals to dissolve the superficial layers of the skin in order to allow for a healthier, more even surface to appear.

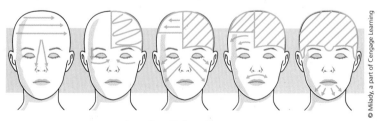

chemical peeling

© Milady, a part of Cengage Learning

chemo-exfoliants—the use of chemicals, as opposed to particulates, to exfoliate the stratum corneum.

chemotherapy—treatment of disease by chemical means; typically associated with cancer.

cherry angiomas—condition characterized by the appearance of small elevated red lesions associated with abnormal proliferation of blood vessels; lesions' occurrence increases with age.

chi (CHEE)—concept originally theorized by the Yellow Emperor of China's Han Dynasty. Also called qi. According to chi, nature has a delicate balance. Illness is considered an imbalance.

chloasma—yellow or brown mispigmentation of the skin, also called melasma. Usually the result of external factors such as pregnancy, radiation, or cancer (or cancer treatment).

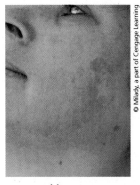

© Milady, a part of Cengage Learning

chloasma

chloracne—form of occupational acne characterized by cysts and pustules resulting from certain chemicals, such as chlorinated hydrocarbons.

chlorine—a highly irritating element; used as a germicide (commonly in the purification of water) and as a bleaching agent.

cholecystitis (koh-lee-sis-TYE-tis)—inflammation of the gall bladder.

cholelithiasis (koh-lee-lih-THIGH-ah-sis)—condition characterized by the formation of gallstones.

cholesterol $C_{27}H_{45}OH$—an alcohol widely found in animal tissues and egg yolks as well as oils and fats. Also found in the brain, spinal cord, liver, kidneys, and adrenal glands. An important component of the body's metabolism in that it is the precursor to steroid hormones such as androgen and estrogen, as well as adrenal corticosteroids. It is well understood that elevated levels of cholesterol are linked to coronary clogging, or coronary heart disease.

cholinergic (koh-luh-NUR-jik)—an agent that produces the parasympathetic muscle effects of acetylcholine at the nerve endings.

chondrus (KON-drus) **crispus**—also known as seaweed, iodine-rich aquatic plant material that aids in thyroid function and is a common ingredient in many preparations including toothpaste, cosmetics, and paints.

chromophore—any chemical in a cell or molecule that is responsible for pigment. In the case of laser therapy, when a molecule absorbs certain wavelengths of visible light, a thermal reaction can occur with resulting damage. A tissue target (chromophore) could be melanin, hemoglobin, water, protein, or dye particles.

chromosome—genetic structure; strands of DNA found in the cell's nucleus.

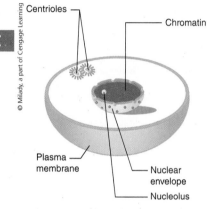

Centrioles

Chromatin

Plasma membrane

Nuclear envelope

Nucleolus

chromosome

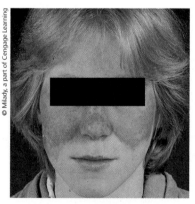

chronic cutaneous lupus erythematosus

chronic—a disease or occurrence showing little or no change over a long period of time.

chronic acid reflux disease—recurrent condition characterized by stomach acids slipping into the esophagus, resulting in a burning sensation in the chest. Also known as GERD.

chronic cutaneous lupus erythematosus (ayr-eh-thee-muh-TOH-sis) **(formerly discoid lupus)**—chronic multisystem disease that mainly affects the skin with rashes and scaling. Typically the skin symptoms are on the face, but they can also be found on the body. The rashes may cause scarring, alopecia, and atrophy.

cinnamates—derivative of cinnaminic acid, it is useful for protection against low levels of UVB rays. Also makes sunscreens waterproof.

cinnamonum zeylanicum (zay-LAN-ee-kum) **(cinnamon oil)**—said to be antimicrobial and antiseptic.

circinate (SUR-suh-nayt)—round.

circuit—route around which an electrical current can flow, beginning and ending at the same point.

circumferential body lift—type of cosmetic surgery for massive weight loss patients that combines buttock lift, outer thigh lift, and tummy tuck, with an incision that runs all the way around the body.

citric acid—alpha hydroxy acid derived from citrus fruit (oranges, grapefruit, etc.).

citrus bergamia (bur-GAY-mee-uh)—herb with antiseptic properties; also called bergamot orange essential oil.

citrus grandis—herb with possible antiseptic properties; also called grape seed oil.

citrus paradise (grapefruit essential oil)—astringent, antiseptic, rich in vitamin C.

clamminess—sensation of the skin feeling cool, damp, moist, and/or sticky to the touch.

claudication—limping due to inadequate blood supply to the legs.

clay—nutrient rich, earth-borne material used in liquids, creams, and face masks; varieties could include bentonite, beetum, and kaolin.

cleansing agents—products that remove foreign matter and secretions from the skin's surface.

cleaving—to split a complex molecule into a similar molecule. Can be accomplished through cell division, chemically or manually.

clinical indication—any sign or circumstance that a particular treatment is appropriate or warranted.

clone—genetically identical cells.

clostridium—any bacteria; anaerobic, spore-forming rod widely found, especially in soil, human intestines, and sometimes in wound infections.

clotting factors—specific proteins that act in sequence to form a clot.

club hair—hair extracted from its root. Presents as rounded or curled.

CO_2 laser—aggressive type of high-power laser used for skin re-surfacing that vaporizes skin and causes thermal injury, allowing for improved collagen production.

coagulation—to clump together.

coal tar—byproduct in coal production used in anti-dandruff shampoos and the treatment of psoriasis. In instances of high exposure, it is also responsible for coal tar acne eruptions of the skin.

cocamide (KOK-uh-mide) **DEA**—agent that increases viscosity for surfactant systems; used in liquid cleansers.

cocamidopropyi betaine (kok-uh-mih-DOP-ihl BEE-tuh-een)—properly called cocamidopropyi dimethyl glycine, this member of the betaine family is used as a mild foaming and cleansing agent to reduce the irritancy of harsher surfactants in shampoos.

cocomonium carbamoylchloride—foaming surfactant with thickening properties.

coccus—bacteria; round or sphere like.

cocos nucifera (KOH-kohs noo-SIF-er-uh)—coconut oil; emollient uses.

coemulisifiers—emulsifiers added to products to stabilize the products' systems.

coenzyme—molecule that is needed for certain enzyme actions; many times it has a vitamin attached.

coenzyme Q10 (ubiquinone)—lipid-soluble cellular antioxidant present in virtually all cells.

cofactors—agents that aid in the functioning of normal processes. Often enzymes or hormones.

cognitive behavioral therapy (CBT)—Type of psychotherapeutic approach that aims to remedy dysfunctional emotions and behaviors through goal-oriented systems aimed at changing the thought processes of affected individuals rather than or in addition to using medications.

coherent light—parallel rays of light that are traveling spatially and temporally in phase with each other.

collagen1—water-soluble protein found in connective tissues. Particularly, type I collagen forms a network in the epidermis, and it is credited with providing skin with its tensile strength and firmness. There are 23 types of collagen in the body.

Collagen2—dermal filler; the trade name for bovine collagen.

collateral circulation—to naturally or medically route circulation around a damaged or diseased artery.

collimated light—a very thin beam of laser light in which all rays run parallel.

color additive—products used to add color to skin care products; iron oxides, FD&C (Federal Food, Drug and Cosmetic Act), D&C,(Drug and Cosmetic approved color) zinc oxides.

color wheel—a circular representation of colors in relation to their closeness to other colors; relevant in makeup application.

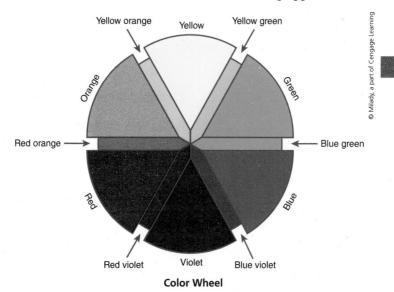

Color Wheel

columella (kol-yuh-MEL-uh)—(1) a miniature column (2) the raised area between the nares and the upper lip. At the upper lip the columella forms the Cupid's bow.

comedo (KOH-meh-doh) **(plural comedones)**— the primary sign of acne, consisting of a dilated hair follicle filled with keratin, bacteria, and sebum. Comedones may be closed or open.

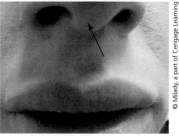

comedogenic—cosmetics or products that cause the skin to become congested and form acne comedones.

comedogenesis—tending to cause or aggravate acne.

columella

comedogenicity—ability to which a product or agent will clog pores.

comedolytic—any agent that prevents acne from occurring.

comfrey extract—used as a healing agent; also has emollient properties.

commiphora myrrha (kom-MEE-for-uh MEER-uh)—antiseptic, antimicrobial, anti-inflammatory; from the myrrh bush.

complications—a difficulty, a complex state, or a disease suffered by an individual without being specifically related, yet affecting the original disease.

compounding—putting together components to create products; usually active ingredients.

computed axial tomography scans (CT scan)—a sectional view of the body shown by computed tomography. Used to diagnose and identify diseases and conditions such as cancer, soft tissue irregularities, and inflammations.

concha (KONG-kuh)—the outer ear.

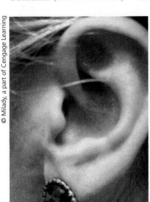
© Milady, a part of Cengage Learning

concha

conductor—a substance that allows electricity to pass through it.

conjunctiva—mucous membrane lining of the eyelids.

conjunctivitis—inflammation of the conjunctiva within the eye.

connective tissue—fibrous tissue that binds, protects, cushions, and supports the various parts of the body.

consent—required clinical documentation in which associated risks, complications, and presumable outcomes are outlined in association with a given procedure. This document gives permission by the patient to the nurse, doctor, or esthetician to provide the procedure.

consequence—a predictable outcome of the procedure that occurs in a reasonable percentage of people having the procedure.

constriction—the process of narrowing.

consultation—initial visit with a professional during which the client and the professional both investigate whether a specific treatment or service is warranted or achievable.

consumer rights and responsibilities—ensures that patients are informed of certain choices including providers and plans, access to emergency services, participation in treatment decisions, respect and nondiscrimination, confidentiality of health information, and complaints and appeals.

contact allergic dermatitis—skin condition characterized by close repeated contact with an allergen or irritant resulting in hives, pruritis, and irritation.

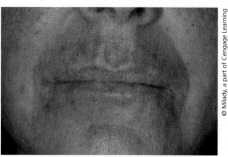

contact allergic dermatitis

© Milady, a part of Cengage Learning

contaminant—an agent that brings a dirty, undesired component into a controlled environment and has the potential to cause harm or injury.

contaminate—the process by which a device or compound becomes nonsterile or impure through contact with another device or compound.

contracture—the replacement of normal elastic tissue with fibrous inelastic skin, in the case of scarring or burns. The affected areas become tight and difficult to move.

contraindication—any sign, condition, or symptom that renders a particular treatment inadvisable, inappropriate, or even dangerous.

converter—device used to switch from alternating current to direct current.

copper—nontoxic; as a trace element in topical preparations, it has a catalytic action for keratinization. May also play a role in the formation of collagen by promoting certain enzymatic activities.

corneal abrasion—a scratch or abrasion on the clear protective tissue on the eye.

corneocytes—cells within the epidermis that act as the "bricks" to the "mortar," or the cement, of intercellular lipids.

cornified—hardening or thickening of the epidermis.

corpus luteum—structure involved in production of progesterone.

corrugator—muscle that draws the eyebrows medially and inferiorly.

cortex—the middle layer; a fibrous protein core formed by elongated cells containing melanin.

corticosteroid—hormonal steroid substances that originate in the adrenal gland and regulate biochemical reactions to occur at prescribed optimal rates.

Corticotrophin releasing hormone (CRH)—neurotransmitter responsible for the brain's stress response.

cortisone—a hormone secreted by the adrenal gland. It is produced by the adrenal gland and manufactured synthetically. In the body it is converted to cortisol, where it is vital in the metabolism of fats, carbohydrates, sodium, and fats. Synthetically, it is used to treat rheumatoid arthritis, allergies, and other maladies.

cosmeceutical—products that do more than decorate or camouflage, but less than prescription drugs would do. The term was originally coined by Dr. Albert Kligman.

cosmetics—*see* applied cosmetics.

cosmetic surgery—any elected surgical procedure, often involving plastic surgery, that is intended to preserve or improve outward appearance.

Cosmoderm—trade name for 3.5% autologous collagen.

Cosmoplast—trade name for 6.5% autologous collagen.

course—the path that a given disease or condition can expect to take under ideal circumstances.

cranial nerve V—also called the trigeminal nerve; provides sensation to the ears, nose, mouth, lower face, and lower eyes (*see* illustration on next page).

cranial nerve VII—also known as the facial nerve; aids in facial movement (*see* illustration on next page).

cross-contamination—undesirable components (bacteria) that move to another material usually through improper handling (such as using the hands rather than a sterile spatula). In skin care, an example is moving product with the fingers from one jar of product into another jar of product.

croton (KROHT-un) **oil**—a fixed oil extracted from the croton plant. Also known as castor oil, it used to be used as a cathartic, but has been proven to be toxic. It is used still as a moisturizing agent in cosmetic preparations.

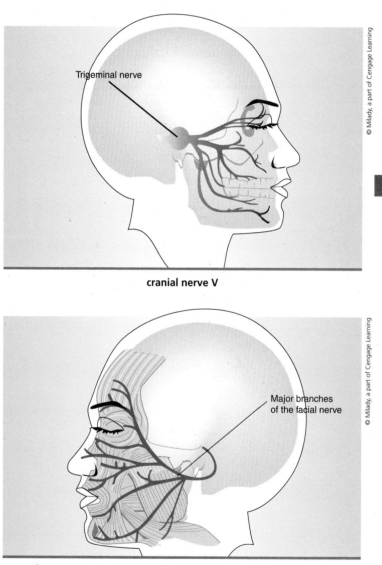

cranial nerve V

cranial nerve VII

crow's feet—dynamic rhytides next to the eyes, caused by repeated muscle movement from expression over time.

crus—resembling a leg.

crust—any dried substance including sebum, blood, and pus.

cryogen—a substance used to produce extremely low temperature; particularly refers to liquid nitrogen.

cryotherapy—treatment modality that uses cold as a means to treat certain cutaneous conditions.

culture—(1) the induced and managed growth of microorganisms for diagnostic purposes (2) the ideas, values, traditions, and symbols of a society.

culture medium—mixture of organic and inorganic products used to grow bacteria or other cells.

curcumin (KUR-kyoo-min)—naturally occurring pigment in the yellow family. It is the pigment that gives the spice tumeric its yellow color.

Cushing Syndrome—named for Harvey Cushing, a U.S. surgeon. A syndrome in which there is excessive secretion of the adrenal cortex. This could be caused by a tumor or hyperfunctioning of the pituitary gland.

cutaneous—pertaining to the skin.

cuticle—a layer of dead epidermal cells; the outermost layer of hair; consisting of one overlapping layer of transparent, scale-like cells around the fingernail.

Cutivate—moderate-strength topical steroid used for inflammation and allergic responses.

cyanosis—bluish-coloring of the skin resulting from reduced levels of oxygen in the blood.

cylindrical—referring to a tubular shape.

cytokines (SYE-toh-kines)—any number of substances that send immunologic signals to or between cells.

cytomegalovirus retinitis (sye-toh-meg-ah-loh-VYE-rus ret-ih-NYE-tis)—viral inflammation of the retina. The virus is present in almost everyone. Typically, it can be fought off, but in immunosuppressed individuals this virus can cause damage to the retina and the rest of the body. Those that are typically at risk include HIV positive, immunosuppressed individuals, and chemotherapy or bone transplant patients.

cytoplasm—fluid contents outside the cell nucleus in which the organelles are suspended.

cytotoxic—poisonous or destructive to cells.

d-alpha tocopherol—*see* Vitamin E.

dandelion extract—herb that is rich in minerals; used as a topical tonic to correct pH.

daucus carota (DOH-kus kar-OH-tuh)—herb that has antioxidant properties; precursor to Vitamin A.

daughter cells—the cells that are the product of cellular meiosis or mitosis of another cell (*see* mitosis).

DEA (diethanolamine)—organic alkali used to neutralize organic acids.

decontamination—the process by which to reduce toxic substances.

decyl (DES-uhl) **alcohol**—anti-foaming agent found in perfumes.

decyl glucoside (DES-ul GLOO-kuh-side)—foaming agent, as in cleansers.

decyl polyglucose (DES-ul pol-ee-GLOO-kohs)—used in cleansers for its foaming factor.

deep epidermal wounding—injury that reaches deep into the epidermis. This wound heals quickly because the appendages are still intact and epidermal cells necessary to wound healing reside in this depth and are readily available to usher in healing processes.

deep peels—peel depth extending into the papillary dermis or upper reticular dermis. Most notable of deep peels is phenol.

deep vein thrombosis—also known as DVT; the formation of abnormal blood clots in the deep veins, typically of the legs. This problem can be life-threatening, and the patient should seek immediate medical attention. Signs and

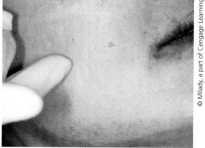

TCA peel (deep peel)

© Milady, a part of Cengage Learning

symptoms include pain, swelling, tenderness, changes in the color of the extremity, and the area will be warm to the touch. Unfortunately, many people do not have symptoms. This is called a "silent" DVT.

de-fatted—also called degrease, process used prior to a peel; the use of isopropyl alcohol or acetone to remove all oils from the skin. This pre-peel technique will allow peel solutions to work evenly.

degree—(1) severity; advanced certification (2) unit of temperature measurement.

dehydrated skin—the result of decreased moisture content in the skin due to decreased sebum output or changes in the natural moisturizing factor or transepidermal water loss of the skin. Dehydrated skin often feels tight, has small pores, and sometimes even has a thin layer of visible dry stratum corneum present.

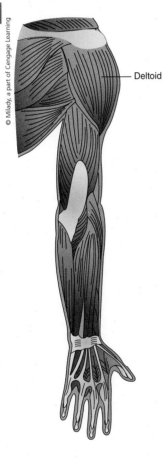

Deltoid

© Milady, a part of Cengage Learning

dehydroepiandrosterone (dee-hye-droh-ep-ee-an-DROS-teh-rohn) **sulfate**—naturally occurring endogenous steroid that is converted into testosterone.

deltoid muscle—triangular muscle found in the upper arm that raises the arms to the side.

demodex folliculorum (DEM-eh-deks fuh-lik-yuh-LOR-um)—parasite that some suggest may play a role in rosacea.

demulcent (deh-MUL-sent)—agent that will soothe or soften the area in which it is applied. Acts on mucous membranes; barley, licorice, and linseed are herbal demulcents.

denatured—alteration of the normal or usual nature of a substance.

deodorant—an agent that masks or absorbs bacterial body odor.

deoxygenate—to deplete the tissues or organs of oxygen.

deoxyribonucleic acid (DNA)—The long double-helix strand of genetic information contained within cells; discovered by Wilkins, Crick, and Watt.

depigment—the loss of normal pigment through peeling or disease.

depilatory—topical agent that destroys surface hair but does not kill the root.

depression—(1) an area of skin that is lower than surrounding tissue (2) condition characterized by low mood; loss of interest and energy; changes in weight, appetite, and sleep patterns; fatigue; the inability to concentrate; feelings of low self-worth; and possibly thoughts of suicide.

depressor supercilli—(soo-per-SIL-ee-eye) muscle of the eye that acts to draw the eyebrow downward.

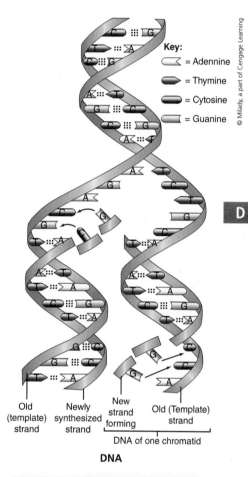

Key:
- ◁ = Adennine
- ● = Thymine
- ◖ = Cytosine
- ◻ = Guanine

Old (template) strand | Newly synthesized strand | New strand forming | Old (Template) strand

DNA of one chromatid

DNA

© Milady, a part of Cengage Learning

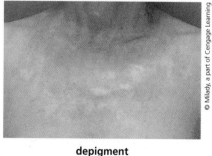

depigment

© Milady, a part of Cengage Learning

depurative (DEP-yuh-ray-tiv)—agent that purifies or cleanses.

dermabrasion—predecessor to microdermabrasion, which used a wire brush or a diamond-coated wheel to resurface the skin to the papillary dermal level.

dermal-epidermal junction (DEJ)—located on the superficial side of the dermis and connected to the basal layer of the epidermis. The DEJ is itself made up of specialized tissue that connects the layers of skin.

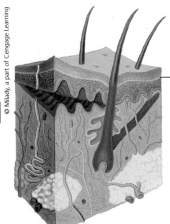

Dermal epidermal junction (DEJ)

dermal filler—general name given to all-natural and synthetic injectables, whose agents act to smooth lines and wrinkles.

dermal papilla—small, cone-shaped indentation at the base of the

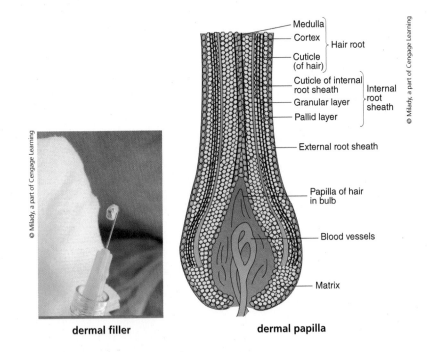

Medulla
Cortex } Hair root
Cuticle (of hair)

Cuticle of internal root sheath
Granular layer } Internal root sheath
Pallid layer

External root sheath

Papilla of hair in bulb

Blood vessels

Matrix

dermal filler   **dermal papilla**

© Milady, a part of Cengage Learning

hair follicle that fits into the hair bulb; also called the hair papilla.

dermal scattering—the change that occurs between the laser's spot size at the surface of the skin and the spot size deeper in the tissue.

dermaplaning—exfoliation of the outer layers of skin (stratum corneum) or vellus hairs with a sharp flat blade.

dermatitis—inflammation of the skin.

dermatofibroma—skin condition characterized by benign nodular tumor growth.

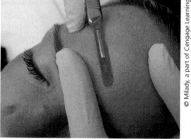

dermaplaning

dermatologic investigation—the process by which a medical professional conducts a visual skin examination of the skin in order to understand the distribution, location, and morphology of the appearance of questionable lesions, rashes,

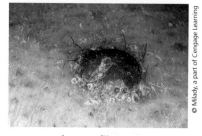

dermatofibroma

or growths in order to diagnose a skin-related condition.

dermatologist—one who is a medical specialist in the area of disease affecting the skin.

dermatome—a delineated area of the skin that follows a nerve route. A dermatome is often seen following shingles.

dermatophyte—any number of fungi which inhabit the skin.

dermis—The second layer of skin (*see* Figure 2.40 on page 56). There are two layers within the dermis: the papillary dermis and the reticular dermis. The papillary dermis is connected to the epidermis, and the reticular dermis is connected to the subcutaneous tissue.

dermodex folliculorum—common, universally distributed parasite that infects the hair follicles; linked to rosacea.

desiccation—removal of all fluids; to dry.

designer peel—custom-made combinations of herbal and prescription ingredients.

desmosomes—small, hairlike structures; cells that are specialized in cell-to-cell adhesion. Common in skin and muscle tissue.

desquamation—exfoliation or shedding of the stratum corneum.

detergent—a synthetic cleansing agent that acts as a wetting agent and emulsifier.

diagnosis—the processes by which medical professionals evaluate, understand, and identify a disease or condition in an individual. The purpose of a diagnosis is to have a reasonable course of treatment and prognosis.

diaphoretic (dye-uh-fuh-RET-ik)—perspiration; agents that promote or increase perspiration.

diastole—part of the normal rhythm of the heart during that the heart chambers expand to fill with blood. Opposite of systole, or contraction.

diathermy (DYE-uh-thur-mee)—therapeutic treatment which uses high-frequency currents to generate heat.

diatomaceous earth—an abrasive agent for cleansers and exfoliates.

dibenzoylmethanes—UVA ray absorber. Used commonly in sunscreens and UV-protecting moisturizers.

diffuse surface reflection—deflection of a ray of light in many directions when it comes in contact with a textured surface, as in the skin; related to the use of laser beams.

diffusion—the movement of molecules from one area to another, typically dependent on the concentration; moving from high concentration to lower concentration. An example of this would be water moving into the lymph system depending on the concentration of salt in the body.

digestives—herbs that assist with digestion; for example, cumin and turmeric.

dilation—the process of widening or expanding an orifice or vessel.

dilution—the process of weakening the concentration.

dimethicone—from silicone; used for lubrication in skin care products.

diminutive—to denote smallness or being smaller than something else.

dioctyl sodium sulfosuccinate (dye-OK-til SOH-dee-um sul-foh-SUK-sih-nayt)—a surfactant.

diopters (dye-AHP-turs)—unit of measurement relating to the power of a lens.

diploid—paired chromosomes; humans have 46 pairs.

diplopia (dih-PLOH-pee-ah)—double vision.

discoid lupus—*see* chronic cutaneous lupus erythematosus.

disinfect—the process by which microbial agents are reduced with heat or chemicals.

disodium EDTA—preservative used in cosmetic preparations.

diuretic—product or agent that will increase urination.

DMDM hydantoin(hye-DAN-toh-in)—safe, widely used preservative.

DNA—*see* deoxyribonucleic acid.

dopamine—neurotransmitter whose performance is associated with many mental disorders. It is also essential to proper central nervous system function.

dopamine agonist—any agent that increases dopamine activity and activates dopamine receptors.

dorsum—the back surface; when relating to the nose, the bridge.

dosage form—the means by which a drug is delivered, whether it be topical, pill, injectible, etc.

double blind test—for clinical trials of a product or during an experiment. The testing parties and subjects are unaware of the critical aspects of the test or experiment until the end of testing.

dowager hump—a bump that forms along the spine due to slow bone loss (osteoporosis) overtime. (Dowager means "dignified elderly woman.") This disease is more common in women than men, though men can get the disease. Also called kyphosis.

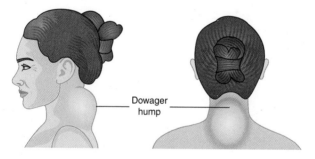

Dowager hump

© Milady, a part of Cengage Learning

drug—products for the cure and treatment of disease or health problems.

drug reaction—unintended and undesirable effects from a drug.

dry heat sterilization—the process of killing bacteria with dry heat rather in an autoclave.

dry skin—a condition resulting from a decrease in sebum production, the natural moisturizing factor (NMF), and an increase in trans-epidermal water loss (TWEL). *See* dehydrated skin.

durability—(1) the wherewithal to withstand a rigorous test (2) refers to the length of time a dermal filler will last.

dynamic conditions—circumstance in which the subject matter is in a state of often unmanageable, constant change.

dynamic movement—the movement of muscles associated with expression; typically facial.

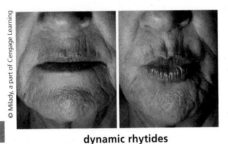

dynamic rhytides (RYE-tides)—wrinkling that occurs in reference to muscle movement.

dyschromia—abnormal and unwanted discoloration of the skin.

dynamic rhytides

dysmorphic—being abnormally formed.

dyspepsia—symptomatic condition characterized by abnormal or painful digestion. Not a disease itself, but symptomatic of other diseases, usually gastric in nature.

dysphagia—condition characterized by difficulty swallowing.

dysphoria—feelings of depression, discomfort, or unhappiness with no known cause.

dysplastic nevus—an atypical morphing mole that could become cancerous.

dyspnea—condition characterized by difficulty breathing. Sometimes accompanied by pain and often associated with rigorous activity.

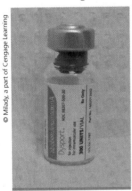

Dysport—trade name for botulism toxin, which is injected into the wrinkle-causing muscles. The toxin blocks the release of acetylcholine, which would otherwise signal the muscle to contract, thus paralyzing the injected muscle. Dysport carries a black box warning. (*See* black box warning.).

dysthymia (dis-THYE-mee-uh)—chronic, mild depression often occurring from secondary antagonists (i.e., side effect from medication).

dystonia (dis-TOH-nee-uh)—abnormality characterized by prolonged, repetitive muscle contractions that may cause twisting or jerking movements of the body part affected.

Dysport

ear reflexology—an ancient Chinese technique that uses pressure-point techniques on the ears to restore the flow of energy throughout the entire body.

eatlah—(e-la) *see* threading.

ecchymosis (ek-ih-MOH-sis)—bruising resulting from blood escaping into the skin of mucous membranes, usually as the result of minor trauma, but may be indicative of a more serious underlying condition.

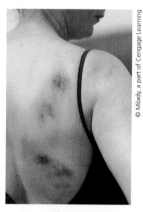

ecchymosis

eccrine (EK-rin) **sweat glands**—smaller of the sweat glands that are distributed over the skin's surface. They are responsible in regulating the body's temperature.

echinacea (ek-ih-NAY-see-uh)—herb derived from the purple coneflower, native to western U.S. Thought to be an antiviral and antibacterial.

E. coli (Escherichia coli)—gram-negative bacteria; fast growing. Commonly found in the GI tract; when outside the GI tract, it will usually cause infections.

eczema—*see* atopic dermatitis.

eczematoid dermatitis (EK-zeh-muh-toyd der-muh-TYE-tis)—form of dermatitis caused by the spreading of purulent material from an infected site.

edema (eh-DEE-muh)—swelling resulting from excessive fluid buildup in tissue. Resulting from a variety of causes ranging from lymphatic obstruction to trauma, it may be indicative of a more serious underlying condition.

EDTA—*see* ethylenediaminetetraacetic acid.

efficacy—(1) achieving the desired result (2) how well a product or treatment works.

effusion—the leakage of a gas or fluid where otherwise sealed.

eflornithine (eh-FLOR-neh-theen)—chemical substance agent that blocks or inhibits hair growth. Known by the trade name Vaniqa, this product is often used on blond or gray hair that is not treatable with a laser.

Efudex (EF-yoo-deks) **(5-FU or fluorouracil)**—antimetabolite used in treating actinic keratosis and certain types of cancer, including superficial basal cell carcinomas. Treatment takes about 2–3 weeks, with the first stage beginning as an inflammatory response followed by a sloughing or scabbing stage. As the skin begins to heal, typically all the actinic keratoses are removed.

elastase (ih-LAS-tayz)—naturally occurring sugar used to convert elastin and other proteins into amino acids; enzyme that destroys elastin.

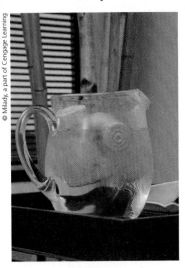

© Milady, a part of Cengage Learning

elastic wraps

elastic wraps—the use of binding bandages around a client's legs in a tight and secure manner; used in the spa to remedy leg fatigue.

elastin—a protein that is a component of connective tissue; usually found in the middle layer of arteries. It is the principal fiber that gives skin its elastic qualities. Used topically in cosmetic preparations for the purpose of moisturizing.

eldopaque (EL-doh-pak)—4% concentration of hydroquinone used as a skin-bleaching agent.

elais guineensis (eh-LAY-us gin-ee-EN-sis) **(palm kernel oil)**—emollient and lubricant used in cosmetic preparations.

electrodesiccation—the destruction of tissue cells with the use of electric sparks; used as a treatment modality for certain cutaneous conditions such as sebaceous hyperplasia.

electrologist—individual skilled in the use of electricity to remove hair; synonymous with electrolysist.

electrology—the general study of electricity, its properties, and its applications.

electrolysis—the use of an electric current to remove moles, warts, or hair roots.

electrolysist—*see* electrologist.

electrolytes—any solution that conducts electricity in the body, most commonly salts, potassium, and chlorine.

electrons—stable, negatively charged elementary particles that orbit the nucleus of an atom.

electrosurgical units (ESU)—any electrical device used for cauterizing or cutting tissue.

electrothermal stimulation—use of heat and light to produce skin regeneration.

elevation—(1) ability to rise vertically (2) used to describe abnormal moles or lesions of the skin.

emetic (eh-MET-ik)—an agent meant to induce vomiting.

EMLA—a popular prescription-required topical anesthetic used by electrolysists and medical professionals; acronym of "eutectic mixture of local anesthetics."

emollient—used in topical cosmetic preparation to help with the smoothness and flexibility of the skin. Often lipids with lubricating action.

emulsification—the mixture of two substances that are not commonly soluble; for instance, oil and water.

emulsifier—a substance that reduces surface tension; used in cosmetic preparations, an agent that binds oil and water ingredients.

emulsion—mixture of soluble oil and water ingredients found in most creams and lotions.

endemic—used to describe a cycle of a mild diseases occurring in a localized population, such as seasonal flu or colds; opposite of epidemic.

endocrine gland—glands that secrete hormones that are carried via blood to specific organs; the pituitary, pancreas, ovaries (females), and testes (males) are endocrine glands.

endocrine system—network of glands and organs that produce hormones.

endocrinologist—one who specializes in the study and treatment of hormones and glands and related diseases.

endometriosis—fairly common disease of the endometrium resulting in tissue buildup outside the uterus.

endometrium—the mucous membrane lining the interior walls of the uterus.

E

endomysium (en-doh-MIZ-ee-um)—thin tissue sheath housing the muscle fibers.

endorphin—polypeptide produced by the brain; creates analgesia.

endoscopy—insertion of a tube with an optical device through an incision or cavity in order to observe an organ or other internal tissues.

endospore—thick-walled spore.

endotoxin—poisonous molecule that is part of gram-negative bacteria and is only released when the bacteria is broken down.

energy fluence—the energy level of a laser; measured in joules.

enzyme—organic catalysts that promote reactions within the body. Virtually all body functions are produced with the assistance of enzymes.

EO—*see* essential oil.

eosinophil (ee-oh-SIN-oh-fil)—granulocyte blood cell characterized by multiform nucleus.

ephelides (eh-FEL-ih-deez)—type of genetic freckling common in people with fair skin. They tend to fade in winter and reappear following repeated UV exposure in warmer months.

epicardium—inner layer of the pericardium that has direct contact with the heart.

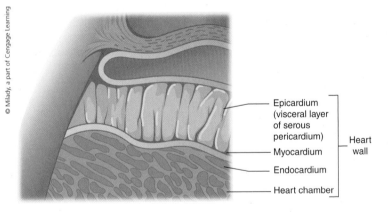

© Milady, a part of Cengage Learning

Epicardium
(visceral layer
of serous
pericardium)

Myocardium

Heart
wall

Endocardium

Heart chamber

epicardium

epidemic—a disease that has the ability to spread rapidly and affect many people over large geographic areas.

epidermal cells—specialized cells which comprise the outermost layer of skin (*see* illustration on next page).

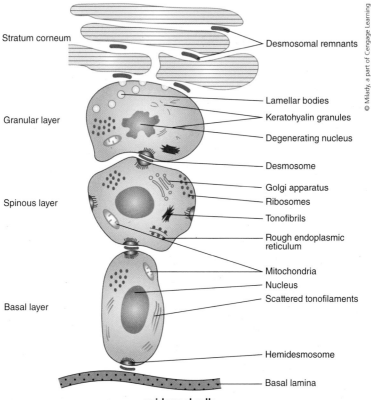

epidermal cells

epidermal cysts—common benign tumors that originate in the epidermis, most often from hair follicles.

epidermal necrosis—destruction of epidermal tissues.

epidermis—the thin, outermost layer of the skin; has five layers. Above the dermis (*See* illustration on next page.)

epidermolysis—separating of the epidermal cells.

epilepsy—neurological disorder involving episodes of abnormal electrical discharge in the brain characterized by seizures, convulsions, and loss of consciousness.

epimysium (ep-ih-MIZ-ee-um)—outer layer of connective tissue sheathing a muscle.

epinephrine (ep-ih-NEF-rin)—hormone that produces the fight or flight response.

epiphora (eh-PIF-oh-ruh)—abnormal excessive or defective flow of tears; obstruction of a tear duct.

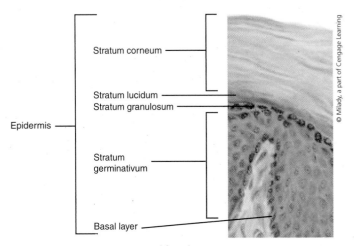

Epidermis

Stratum corneum

Stratum lucidum
Stratum granulosum

Stratum
germinativum

Basal layer

© Milady, a part of Cengage Learning

epidermis

epithelialization—the growth of new skin over a wound.

epithelial tissue—the tissue that forms a thin protective layer on bodily surfaces.

epithelium—cells that make up the top layer of skin; the surface of membranous tissue covering internal organs and lining skin appendages.

epsom salts—magnesium sulphate used for detoxifying; most often used in therapeutic baths.

erbium laser—moderately aggressive type of laser that causes less injury to the deep dermis, while still causing epidermal and papillary dermal injuries.

erector spinae (SPEE-nuh)—long muscle that spans the length of the back and neck. Key component to upright posturing.

ergonomic—physically compatible with body contouring as to prevent or limit long-term joint damage associated with repeated use; ergonomically correct.

ergot (UR-gut) **medicines**—classification of drugs primarily used to treat migraine headaches.

erosion—(1) gnawing away (2) superficial loss of epidermal tissue.

erosive esophagitis—condition characterized by the eroding of the esophagus, possibly resulting in ulceration; most commonly caused by chronic acid reflux disease.

eruptive—pertaining to a breakout on the skin.

erythema (ayr-ih-THEE-muh)—an area or spot on the skin showing diffused redness. It is most often caused by capillary congestion.

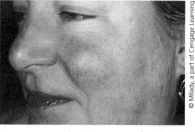

erythema

erythema multiforme (ayr-ih-THEE-muh mul-teh-FOR-mee)—condition characterized by macular eruptions in a patchy formation on the extremities. Etiology is unknown.

erythema nodosum (ayr-ih-THEE-muh noh-DOH-sum)—characterized by tender, red bumps, usually found on the shins. Quite often, erythema nodosum is not a separate disease but, rather, a sign of some other disease, or of sensitivity to a drug.

erythrocyte (eh-RITH-roh-site)—red blood cell manufactured in the bone marrow; has hemoglobin-carrying oxygen.

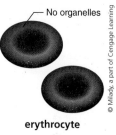

No organelles

erythrocyte

erythrocyte sedimentation rate—the rate at which red blood cells enter into the bloodstream in a one-hour period.

essential fatty acid—a fatty acid that cannot be supplied by the body; must be found in the diet.

essential hypertension—high blood pressure without a known cause.

essential oil—botanical origins achieved through steam distillation or mechanical expression. Used therapeutically at home in many cosmetic and therapeutic remedies or in the clinic or spa for medicinal or therapeutic preparations.

ester—a fragrant water and fat-soluble compound formed by the combination of an organic acid and alcohol, removing the water from the compound.

estradiol (es-truh-DYE-ol)—the so-called pregnancy hormone. Produced by the ovaries and excreted in the urine of pregnant women.

estrogens—group of hormones responsible for secondary sex characteristics in women.

ethanol—*see* ethyl alcohol.

ethyl alcohol—a colorless flammable liquid with a fruity smell produced by fermentation; often used as a solvent; synonymous with ethanol; grain alcohol.

ethylenediaminetetraacetic (ETH-uh-leen-DYE-uh-meen-TEH-truh-uh-SEE-tik) **acid (EDTA)**—chelating agent that augments a formulation's preservative system.

etiologic (ee-tee-uh-LOJ-ik) **agent**—substance or organism that causes disease.

etiology (ee-tee-OL-oh-jee)—the study of origins and/or causes of conditions and diseases.

eucalyptus oil—antiseptic, disinfectant; used originally by the Aborigines; may cause allergic responses.

eumelanin (yoo-MEL-uh-nin)—the darkest and most pure, often brown to black, tones of melanin associated with skin and hair coloration.

euphoria—emotional state of excitement, well-being, and happiness.

eutectic (yoo-TEK-tik) **mixture**—a mixture of two or more agents with a lower melting point than any of the individual agents.

exanthema (eg-san-THEE-muh)—any inflamed skin eruptions; for example, a widespread rash.

excipient—a neutral carrier for the active ingredients in pharmacological or cosmetic ingredients.

excited states—the conditions of a physical system in which the energy level is higher than the lowest possible level.

excoriation—linear erosion caused by mechanical means and resulting in epidermal abrasion.

excretion—the act of discharging waste matter from tissues or organs.

exfoliate—to remove surface dead skin cells with the use of an abrasive agent such as synthetic or natural grains, revealing a fresh and glowing skin tone.

exfoliating treatments—any therapeutic treatment intended to remove surface dead skin cell with the use of an abrasive agent, synthetic or natural grains, enzymes, or chemicals, revealing a fresh and glowing skin tone.

exocrine—secreting externally through a gland, reaching the epidermal surface; opposite endocrine.

exotoxins—a toxic substance created by microorganisms and released into surrounding tissue.

expiration date—the date after which a product or drug should not be used; end of product's shelf life.

expression—technique used for extracting the essential oils from citrus products; for example, cold pressing.

extensor digitorum longus—thin, long muscle of the lower leg; responsible for extending the four smallest toes and pronating the foot.

external—outside; opposite internal.

external obliques—outermost layer of muscle tissue lining the abdomen.

external root sheath—the inner side of the follicular canal which is made of horny cells.

extrapyramidal—existing outside of the pyramidal tracts of the central nervous system. Important in muscle tone and equilibrium.

extrinsic aging—changes which are brought on by the effects of the environment and our choices relating to them, specifically sun exposure.

exudate (EG-soo-dayt)—(1) pus or sebum that oozes out (2) fluid with a high concentration of protein and cellular debris that has escaped from blood vessels and has been deposited in or on tissue, usually from infection (pus).

eyelashes—hairs found on the tip of the eyelid whose physiologic purpose is to block debris from getting into the eye.

eyelids—thin vascular layers of skin whose physiologic purpose is to block sweat and debris from getting into the eye.

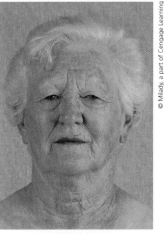

extrinsic aging

© Milady, a part of Cengage Learning

E

F

F—abbreviation for Fahrenheit degrees of temperature measurement.

facelift—surgical lifting of facial skin and muscles below to create a younger appearance.

facial—generic name for a treatment that applies agents intended to cleanse, tone, purify, stimulate, and/or calm the skin on the face.

facial reflex—contraction of the middle face muscle when the eyes are touched.

facilitated diffusion—a process of molecule movement that occurs with the assistance of proteins that act as carriers.

faculative anerobes (FAK-ul-tay-tiv AN-uh-rohbs)—organisms that live well with or without oxygen.

fango—the Italian word for "mud"; a gray-brown claylike compound mixed with thermal water that is rich in salt, bromine, and iodine and a number of other organic components, such as algae and protozoa. This nutrient-rich mud is spread on the skin and wrapped to allow the nutrients to penetrate for therapeutic purposes.

farnesol—a bioactivator; a component of Vitamin K. Found in lilac, lily of the valley, and sandalwood; used in cosmetic preparations.

fascia (FASH-ee-ah)—a sheet of connective tissue that supports or separates muscles. It connects the skin to the underlying tissue. It can be superficial, allowing free movement of the skin or deep connecting and binding muscles.

fat transfer—process by which fat is taken from one area of the body and used as a dermal filler in another region. Typically fat is taken from the abdomen or hips and used in the nasolabial folds or marionette lines to correct facial aging.

fatty acid—any of a large group of basic acids; saturated or unsaturated. Important for maintaining healthy skin and necessary for human life. Most are taken in through the diet. They would be insoluble if not for salts in bile that enable absorption.

FDA—*see* Food and Drug Administration.

femoral vein—deep vein which runs down each leg alongside of the femur, the long bone of the upper leg.

fennel extract—antiseptic; detoxifier used for oily skin.

fibrillin (FYE-bril-in)—a protein of the connective tissues. It is found in the skin, ligaments, tendons, and in the aorta. Necessary component to wound healing.

fibrin (FYE-brin)—a plasma filament protein that, when combined with fibrogen, is the basis for blood clotting.

fibrinogen—protein present in the blood that is converted to fibrin by calcium ions. Necessary for blood clotting.

fibroblasts—a cell that produces connective tissue; collagen, elastin, reticular proteins.

fibularis muscle group—group of muscles which span the length of the fibula in the lower legs.

filaggrin (fil-AG-grin)—synthesizes lipids (fats) that are thought to serve as intercellular cement in the epidermis; important component of natural moisturizing factor (NMF).

filiform—(1) hairlike in shape (2) in cultures, a growth that is a uniform line. Relevant in the description of certain types of warts.

fissure—cracked or split tissue.

fistulas (FIS-tyoo-lahs)—long, narrow ulcers of unknown etiology.

Fitzpatrick skin typing—method of skin typing that considers skin's complexion, hair color, eye color, and the individual's reaction to unprotected sun exposure. The most common type of skin analysis in the medical spa and medical office.

flash injury—a tissue injury caused by a sudden and rapid exposure to electricity, heat, cold, or chemicals.

flatulence—excessive gas expelled by a body orifice.

flavonoid—naturally occurring pigments often found in plants.

Fleming, Alexander—Scottish physician and researcher who first discovered the ability of mold to kill bacteria.

flexation—the ability of a muscle or muscle group to bend a limb at a central joint.

F

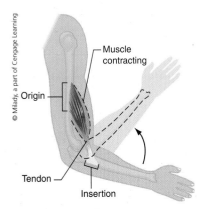

Muscle contracting

Origin

Tendon

Insertion

flexor

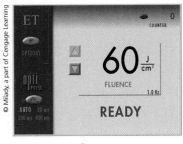

fluence

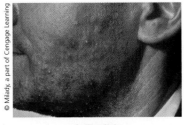

folliculitis

flexor—the major muscle or muscle group which brings two bones close together.

fluence—the measure of radiation (joules/cm^2).

fluid injection liposuction—type of liposuction during which fluids containing lidocaine and other medications and fluids are injected into fatty tissues prior to fat removal.

fluoride—inorganic substance added to toothpaste and water sources to prevent tooth decay.

Fluorouracil (flor-uh-YOOR-uh-sil)—*see* Efudex.

Foley, Howard—researcher who is credited with discovering the medicinal use of penicillin.

folic acid—component of Vitamin B complex; occurs naturally in green plants, liver, and yeast. Has a role in preventing certain birth defects.

follicle—a small sac; for example, when discussing the skin and its appendages, a term used is hair follicle, which contains the hair root and sweat gland.

follicular canal—depression in the skin which encapsulates the pilosebaceous unit.

folliculitis (foh-lik-yoo-LYE-tis)—condition characterized by inflammation of the hair follicles resulting in "ingrown hairs."

Food and Drug Administration (FDA)—regulatory agency of the federal government which oversees food and drugs currently on the market and approves drugs for consumption.

foot reflexology—an ancient Chinese technique that uses pressure-point massage on the feet to restore the flow of energy throughout the entire body.

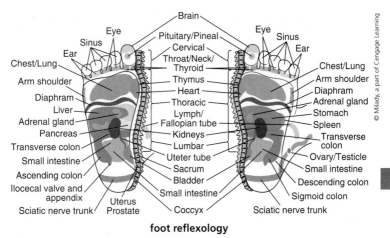

Brain
Eye
Sinus
Ear
Chest/Lung
Arm shoulder
Diaphram
Liver
Adrenal gland
Pancreas
Transverse colon
Small intestine
Ascending colon
Ilocecal valve and appendix
Sciatic nerve trunk
Uterus
Prostate
Pituitary/Pineal
Cervical
Throat/Neck/Thyroid
Thymus
Heart
Thoracic
Lymph/Fallopian tube
Kidneys
Lumbar
Uteter tube
Sacrum
Bladder
Small intestine
Coccyx
Eye
Sinus
Ear
Chest/Lung
Arm shoulder
Diaphram
Adrenal gland
Stomach
Spleen
Transverse colon
Ovary/Testicle
Small intestine
Descending colon
Sigmoid colon
Sciatic nerve trunk

foot reflexology

© Milady, a part of Cengage Learning

foramina (fuh-RAM-uh-nuh)—natural opening through a bone or membrane; typically a passage for nerves and blood vessels.

formaldehyde—used as an antimicrobial agent and a preservative; a possible carcinogenic substance; has a strong odor and is colorless.

formed elements—the red or white blood cells or platelets separated from the fluid part of the blood.

formula—a detailed recipe; specifically relating to the preparation of a medication or, in chemistry, the symbolic expression of the molecules.

fossa—a depression in an organ, organ cavity, or bone.

Four Humors—early medical concept originally documented by Hippocrates, which states

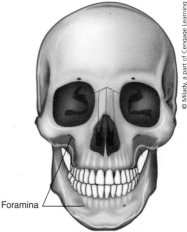

Foramina

© Milady, a part of Cengage Learning

F

that the character of a man was determined by the specific balance of the four fluids (he perceived as) running through the body: black bile, yellow bile, blood, and phlegm.

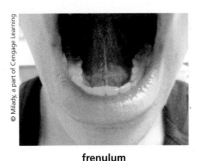

frenulum

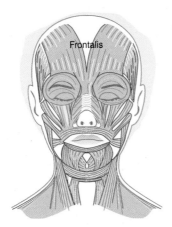

Frontalis

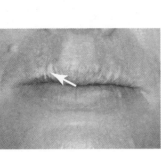

frost

free radicals—come in the form of a single atom or a group of atoms that has at least one unpaired electron. This unpaired electron results in a highly unstable and highly reactive molecule, which tries to gain electrons from neighboring molecules, perpetuating a chain or cascading effect. Damage from free radicals is thought to have great consequence on the skin. Antioxidants reverse free radical damage and are common in esthetic preparations.

frenulum(FREN-yuh-lum)— a small connective tissue that connects a mucous membrane to surrounding tissue; for example, the piece of tissue that connects the tongue to the floor of the mouth.

frontalis (fron-TAY-lis)— muscle which makes up the forehead. Moves the skin of the forehead horizontally and assists with frowning.

frost—(1) deposits of frozen vapor (2) peels associated with changes in skin color and texture, resulting from peel depth. Peels that frost coagulate protein and turn the skin white.

fructose—naturally occurring sugar (e.g., fruits, vegetables).

fruit scrubs—usually refer to a mixture of an exfoliating granule and may contain an alpha-hydroxy acid used as an exfoliation product. They work by dissolving the cellular cement that holds dead skin cells together, revealing a smoother, more even skin tone and promoting an increased cellular turnover.

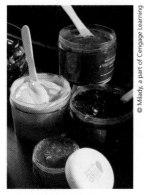

fruit scrubs

full-thickness wound—a wound that penetrates into the papillary dermis or upper reticular dermis. They are associated with slower healing and scarring will typically develop, especially if the wound is in the reticular dermis.

fungal infection—any infection caused by the kingdom of organisms which includes yeasts and molds.

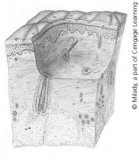

full-thickness wound

fungicide—a product or medication which kills fungi.

fungistatic—a product that inhibits the growth of fungi.

fungus—an organism that belongs to the yeast, mold, or mushroom kingdom.

furuncle (FYOO-rung-kul)—a boil on the skin that is acute and presents with deep inflammation and pus.

fuse—an electrical safety device that contains a piece of metal that will melt if the current running through it exceeds a certain level.

Galen, Claudius—protégé of Hippocrates who is credited with reviving and spreading his teachings.

galvanic electrolysis—the only method of permanent hair removal. Using direct current, the hair follicle is destroyed at the papilla. Direct current (DC) is inserted into the hair follicle while the client holds the power source on the positive side. When the power is applied, the saline in the hair follicle turns to sodium hydroxide, chlorine, and hydrogen gas, thus destroying the follicle.

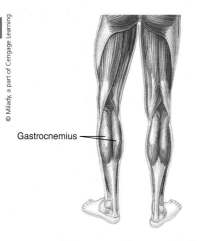

Gastrocnemius

gastrocnemius (gas-trok-NEE-mee-us)—commonly called the "calf" muscle, it is responsible for plantar flexing of the foot and flexing of the knee.

gel solutions—semisolid material which is easily absorbed in the skin without the irritation associated with liquid solutions.

gene—basic unit of heredity; contains DNA. Each gene resides on a specific location on a chromosome, and they are classified as being dominant or recessive depending on their likelihood of being passed on to future generations or not. In special circumstances, a gene can mutate, resulting in variable characteristics from one generation to the next, inasmuch as genetic mutations are responsible for the variation that exists from one individual to the next.

generalized anxiety disorder (GAD)—condition characterized by nonspecific anxiety which develops to the point that it compromises the quality of life for the affected individual.

generalized post-traumatic dyschromias—pigment change associated with tissue injury. Also known as post-inflammatory hyperpigmentation (PIH).

generic drug—a drug without patent protection that is made and advertised under the chemical name; for example, ibuprofen as opposed to Advil.

genetic diseases—diseases that present in genetic material and are passed down through generations. Most genetic diseases begin as mutations and are passed down. They are recessive or dominant, depending on the likelihood that they will be passed down.

genetic engineering—to change the genes by technological means.

genetics—study of heredity; the understanding of how traits are passed from one generation to the next.

germicidal lamps—ultraviolet radiation that kills bacteria, viruses, and fungi.

germicide—any agent which destroys microorganisms.

germinal cells—pertaining to cell reproduction, a cell from which other cells are derived; the cells of the basal layer that reproduce the skin.

gingivial hypoplasia—underdevelopment of the gum tissue.

glabella (gluh-BEL-uh)—area between the eyebrows, whose underlying muscle groups cause creasing, or "frown lines," as a result of repeated squinting or frowning over time.

glabellar—pertaining to the glabella.

Glogau (Gloh-gow)—classification of aging analysis; a system of photoaging analysis which calculates the severity of aging-related damage and assigns a numerical "typing" (type I being mild to type IV being severe). The Glogau classification considers both intrinsic and extrinsic aging factors.

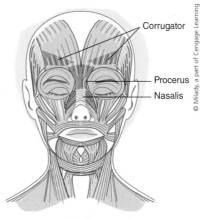

glabella

G

glucagons (GLOO-kah-gons)—hormones secreted by the pancreas that have the ability to increase blood glucose levels.

glucocorticoids—secreted by the adrenal glands, these cortical hormones protect the body against stress and act on the metabolism of the body. The most important glucocorticoid is cortisol.

glucose—simple sugar required for normal metabolism; the most important carbohydrate in the body's energy metabolism.

glucose glutamate—used in hand creams and lotions; humectant.

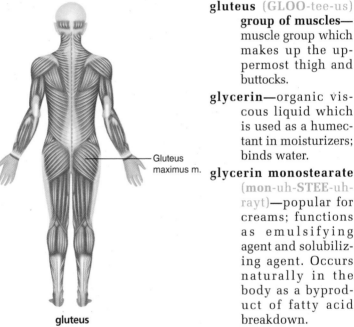

© Milady, a part of Cengage Learning

Gluteus maximus m.

gluteus

gluteus (GLOO-tee-us) **group of muscles**—muscle group which makes up the uppermost thigh and buttocks.

glycerin—organic viscous liquid which is used as a humectant in moisturizers; binds water.

glycerin monostearate (mon-uh-STEE-uh-rayt)—popular for creams; functions as emulsifying agent and solubilizing agent. Occurs naturally in the body as a byproduct of fatty acid breakdown.

glycerol ester—a refined rosin product that can be mixed with honey to produce a wax-like substance.

glycoceramides—glycerin-based lipids which may replace lost intercorneal lipids; helps the skin to bind water, mostly used in lip balms.

glycocitrates—combination of glycolic acid and citric acids; meant for skin that is sensitive or unable to tolerate glycolic acids.

glycolic acid—alpha-hydroxy acid derived from sugarcane, now prepared synthetically. It has a small molecular size that allows for easier penetration into the skin. Used in gels, creams, and peel solutions, as well as exfoliating products. Glycolic acid can be used to improve the skin's tone and texture. It has minimal effects on deep wrinkles and lines, acne scarring or other deep dermal defects. Glycolic acid is found as a peeling product to use in the spa or clinic and as an at-home preparation. It works primarily on the stratum corneum of the skin. It reacts to the skin, causing a loosing of the stratum corneum and a stimulation of cellular growth.

glycoproteins—a group of conjugated proteins that contain a carbohydrate. Many hormones are glycoproteins.

glycosaminoglycans (GAGs)—moisture building polysaccharide chains, most prominent in the dermis, that bind with water; they smooth and soften the surface from below. The most abundant GAG is hyaluronic acid.

glycyrrhizic (glis-eh-RYE-zik) **acid**—derived from licorice root and possessing both anti-inflammatory and antibacterial properties.

gm—gram; a unit of weight measurement.

goiter (GOY-ter)—an enlargement of the thryroid gland, possibly due to a lack of iodine in the diet.

golgi bodies—also called the golgi apparatus. Named after the Italian physician Camillo Golgi. It is responsible for putting together and processing proteins and lipids after synthesis and before they are sent to the endpoint

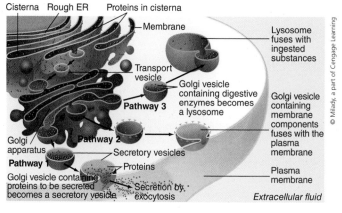

golgi bodies

for use. They are small particles responsible for some enzyme secretion. The golgi body is found in nearly all cells near the nucleus.

gonadotropic—(1) pertaining to the male or female sex organs in the embryonic stage (2) general hormone secreted into the blood that has a specific impact on the sex organs.

grade I acne—acne vulgaris with open and closed comedones with transitory blemishes.

grade II acne—acne vulgaris with larger open and closed comedones, a small number of pustules and papules.

grade III acne—acne vulgaris with many open and closed comedones, pustules, and papules, several cystic lesions, pigment changes, and inflammation, erythema (redness), and area is painful.

grade IV acne—acne vulgaris, which includes all of the above combined with advanced stages of cystic acne, scarring, inflammation, and erythema (redness).

grand mal—a serious seizure associated with epilepsy in which there is loss of consciousness and severe convulsions.

granulocyte (GRAN-yoo-loh-site)—white blood cells involved in immune response; includes neutrophils, eosinophils, and basophils.

granulocytopenia (gran-yoo-loh-sye-toh-PEE-nee-uh)—abnormally low levels of granulocytes in the blood.

granuloma (gran-yoo-LOH-mah)—tumor or inflammatory response produced when the body fails to destroy foreign body product or mycobacteria.

GRAS—acronym for generally recognized as safe.

great saphenous (suh-FEE-nus) **veins**—two veins; one runs deep and the length of the leg, and the other is more superficial. The smaller saphenous vein runs from the foot to the back of the knee and connects with the popliteal vein; it is clearly noticeable on the back of the leg (*see* illustration on next page).

ground state—the condition in which energy in the body or a device is at a low level.

ground substance—consists mainly of glycosaminoglycans (hyaluronic acid, chondroitin sulfate, and dermatan sulfate); involved in maintenance and repair of dermis and other structures as well.

guar hydroxypropyltrimonium (gwar hye-DROK-see-proh-pil-trye-MOH-nee-um) **chloride**—cleansing agent with

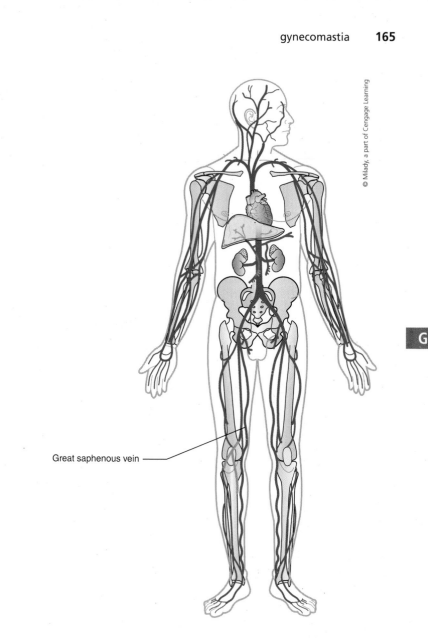

Great saphenous vein ——

© Milady, a part of Cengage Learning

anti-inflammatory, anti-irritant properties commonly used in shampoo formulations; may have skin-softening capabilities.

gynecomastia (guy-neh-koh-MAS-tee-ah)—development of abnormally large breasts in men, which may secrete milk.

hair follicle—*see* follicle.

hair matrix—the germinating center of the hair follicle where mitotic activity occurs.

hallucinations—symptom in which an individual sees or hears things which are not actually there. It is often indicative of psychosis or other severe mental disorders or ingestion of certain substances, called hallucinogenics.

hallucinogenic—an agent which causes temporary hallucination not associated with mental impairment.

hamamelis (ham-uh-MEE-lis)—also called Virginia witch hazel; used as an astringent.

hammam (huh-MOM)—a Turkish bath or steam bath.

hamstrings—group of tendons at the rear of the knee.

hand and foot syndrome (HFS)—also called palmar-plantar erythrodysesthesia or PPE, it is a condition characterized by painful lesions on the hands and feet. It is a result of some types of chemotherapy and some medicines used to treat breast cancer.

hand reflexology—an ancient Chinese technique that uses pressure-point massage on the hands to restore the flow of energy throughout the entire body.

hantavirus pulmonary syndrome (HPS)—a virus that is transmitted to humans through rodent urine and feces with potentially fatal consequences.

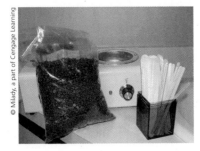

© Milady, a part of Cengage Learning

hard wax—depilatory wax used without a strip.

harvesting—separating cells for regeneration or implantation elsewhere.

hazardous substance—any material which is dangerous; flammable, toxic, or poisonous.

hard wax

healing baths—water treatments to address skin conditions, or joint, muscle, or stress-related disorders.

health hazard—any condition in which exposure may cause chronic health problems or damage to body systems.

Health Insurance Portability and Accountability Act of 1996 (HIPAA)—federal regulation which dictates procedural protocols to protect patient privacy in a medical setting.

health screening—a consultation, a written and verbal process that clears the client for treatment or excludes him or her from treatment due to contraindications.

heart disease—any condition which impairs the normal function of the heart and heart vessels. Typically, angina, myocardial infarction, and arrhythmias are considered heart diseases.

heat—a form of energy.

hectorite—thickening agent.

helicobacter pylori (hel-ih-koh-BAK-tur pye-LOR-ee)—bacteria found in the stomachs of many individuals, thought to be linked to ulcers and stomach cancer.

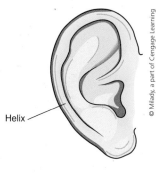

Helix

© Milady, a part of Cengage Learning

H

helix—(1) a coil; pertains to the external ear (2) a conformation of biological polymers.

hematuria (hee-mah-TOO-ree-ah)—blood in the urine.

hemifacial—one side of the face.

hemochromatosis (hee-mah-kroh-mah-TOH-sis)—a hereditary disease in which the body stores more iron than needed, causing the skin to appear bronze. Left untreated, hemochromatosis can lead to organ failure.

hemoglobin—the protein that is housed within the red blood cell that carries the oxygen. Hemoglobin plays a role in the shape of the red blood cell.

hemolytic anemia (hee-moh-LIT-ik ah-NEE-mee-ah)—condition associated with abnormal, premature destruction, breakdown, and removal of red blood cells.

hemophilia (hee-moh-FILL-ee-ah)—recessive genetic disorder occurring almost exclusively in men and boys in which the blood clots much more slowly than normal, resulting in extensive bleeding from even minor injuries.

hemopoietic (hee-moh-poy-ET-ik)—pertaining to the formation of blood cells or blood.

hemoptysis (hee-MOP-tih-sis)—coughing up bloody sputum from respiratory tract or lungs.

hemosiderin (hee-moh-SID-er-in)—coming from hemoglobin; an iron rich pigment that contains iron from deteriorating red blood cells.

HEPA (high efficiency particulate air) filter—smoke evacuator filters that block airborne contaminants down to a 0.3-micron particulate size with 99.9999% efficiency.

heparin (HEP-ah-rin)—polysaccharide that prevents the conversion of thrombin and prothrombin, preventing blood clotting.

hepatitis—inflammation of the liver, commonly thought of as caused by viruses defined as types A, B, or C. Chronic or acute inflammation of the liver can be caused from drugs, alcohol, bacteria, parasites, and chemicals.

hepatotoxin—substance that is destructive to the liver cells.

herb wraps—therapeutic spa treatment which uses a fabric soaked in an herbal tea prior to application to the face or body.

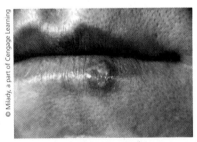

© Milady, a part of Cengage Learning

herpes simplex

herpes simplex virus (HSV)—infectious skin condition characterized by thin-walled vesicles which tend to occur repeatedly in the same place on the skin's surface, usually on mucous membranes or conjunctiva.

herpes zoster—virus responsible for both shingles and chickenpox.

heterogeneous bone grafting—use of a different person's or animal's skeletal material to repair damage to bone and bone structures of another.

heterologous—derived from a different species than the one it is implanted into; such as bovine collagen implanted into humans.

heterotrophs—organism requiring complex foods such as carbohydrates and lipids to grow and develop.

HIPAA—*see* Health Insurance Portability and Accountability Act.

Hippocrates—Greek physician and "father of medicine," who wrote the Hippocratic Oath and the Four Humors.

Hippocratic Oath—ethical oath taken by all doctors relative to the practice of medicine; created by Hippocrates.

hirsutism (HER-soot-izm)—abnormal or unusual hair growth on body parts normally having only downy or vellus hair, i.e., face, arms, and legs of women.

histamine—found in all animal and human cells, this substance is derived from amino acids and produced by basophils and mast cells. Histamine is released via the body's immune system in response to allergens.

HIV—*see* Human Immunodeficiency Virus (HIV).

Hodgkin's disease—uncommon cancer of the lymphatic system, accounts for less than 1% of all cancers in the United States. Other cancers of the lymphatic system are called non-Hodkgin's lymphomas.

holistic—pertinent to the belief that entities are whole and cannot be limited to the function of their parts; use of natural remedies to cure disease.

homomenthyl salicylate (hoh-moh-MEN-thel sal-ih-SIL-ayt)—component of some sunscreens; absorbs UVB.

hormone—synthesized in a gland or organ and sent through the blood as a messenger to another body part in order to inhibit or stimulate metabolic activities.

hormone replacement therapy—therapeutic replacement of hormones as a means to counter the side effects of their absence.

hot spot—areas which will absorb peeling solutions quickly, resulting in a tissue injury.

human gene therapy—the insertion of genetic material into cells to correct a genetic defect.

human genome—the full map of genes for human reproduction.

Human Immunodeficiency Virus (HIV)—virus responsible for Acquired Human Immunodeficiency Syndrome (AIDS). Found in the blood and genital secretions of all individuals who test positive. The disease is spread when the contaminated secretions come in contact with the blood, mucus membranes, or an open cut of another individual. The most common methods of spreading the disease are through sexual contact, sharing needles, and by transmission from infected mothers to their newborns during pregnancy, labor, or breast-feeding.

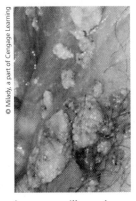

human papillomavirus

human papillomavirus (HPV)—virus responsible for warts. There are over 100 different types of warts that have been identified. The most common warts are the simple warts that individuals get on the hands and feet and genital warts. Genital warts transmitted through sexual activity have been suspected of causing a number of cancers.

humectant—an agent for retaining moisture.

hyaluronic (HYE-eh-loo-ron-ik) **acid**— a glycosaminoglycan found in connective tissue, epithelial tissue, and neural tissues. Used in creams, lotions, and serums as a moisturizing agent.

hydantoin (hye-DAN-toh-in) **anti-convulsants**—drugs which are most commonly used in the treatment of seizures associated with epilepsy.

hydrating facial—restores moisture to the skin and is beneficial for dehydrated skin types.

hydrocarbon—a molecule that is made of hydrogen and carbon; usually found as propellants in aerosols.

hydrocollators—heating units that heat the wrapping linens to an optimal temperature.

hydrogen peroxide—a weak acid that oxidizes quickly. Used as a disinfectant and antiseptic.

hydrolysis—a common process whereby water and salt produce a product with an acid and a base. A common occurrence of hydrolysis is the conversion of protein to amino acids in the digestive process.

hydrolyzed mucopolysaccharides (myoo-koh-pol-ee-SAK-uh-rides)—have properties which assist with TEWL.

hydroquinone (hye-droh-kwih-NOHN)—topical bleaching agent; inhibits the production of tyrosine within melanocytes.

hydrostatic pressure—means of devising fluid pressure by measuring the pressure imposed by an external force.

hydrotherapy—use of chemically or thermally treated water in aesthetic and/or medicinal treatments.

H

hyperacidity—condition in which the body produces too much acid.

hypercalcemia (hye-per-kal-SEE-mee-uh)—high blood calcium.

hyperchloremic acidosis (hye-per-kloh-REE-mik as-ih-DOH-sis)—condition characterized by increased chlorine levels, resulting in higher acidity levels overall.

hypercholesterolemia (hye-per-koh-les-ter-ol-EE-mee-uh)—condition characterized by abnormally high levels of cholesterol in the blood.

hyperchloremia (hye-per-kloh-REE-mee-uh)—high chloride in the blood.

hyperextension—extension of a bodily joint beyond the normal range of motion.

hyperglycemia—increased blood sugar levels that can lead to diabetic coma if unresolved.

hyperinsulinemia (hye-per-in-soo-lin-EE-mee-uh)—condition characterized by excessive levels of insulin in the bloodstream.

hyperkalemia (hye-per-kuh-LEE-mee-uh)—abnormally high levels of potassium in the blood.

hyperkeratosis—thickened areas of the horny layers of skin, particularly the palmar and plantar areas.

hyperlipidemia (hye-per-lip-ih-DEE-mee-uh)—abnormally high levels of fat in the blood.

hyperostosis—excessive bone growth associated with SAPHO.

hyperplasia—excessive proliferation of normal cells in tissue.

hypersensitivity—a circumstance in which the skin overreacts to a product or set of conditions. Presents in a multitude of ways including redness, hives, and pruritis.

hypertension—high blood pressure.

hypertonic solutions—a substance that has higher osmotic pressure than another.

hypertrichosis—excessive hair growth seen in regions of or throughout the body. Can be traced to genetic origin.

hypertrophic scar—overly developed scar tissue

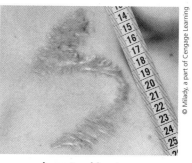

hypertrophic scar

© Milady, a part of Cengage Learning

H

that rises above the skin level, often overfed by an abundance of capillaries. May regress over time.

hyperuricemia (hye-per-yoo-ris-EE-mee-uh)—abnormally high levels of uric acid in the blood.

hypnotic—tending to produce sleep or hypnosis.

hypoallergenic—products that are unlikely to cause skin irritation.

hypocalcemia (hye-poh-kal-SEE-mee-uh)—abnormally low levels of calcium in the blood.

hypodermis—layer of subcutaneous fat and connective tissue lying beneath the dermis.

hypoglycemia (hye-poh-glye-SEE-mee-uh)—abnormally low levels of glucose in the blood.

hypogonadism—condition characterized by underdevelopment of the sexual organs and secondary sexual characteristics.

hypokalemia (hye-poh-kuh-LEE-mee-uh)—abnormally low levels of potassium in the blood.

hypomagnesemia—abnormally low levels of magnesium in the blood, accompanied by muscle irritability.

hypopigmentation—lack of pigmentation in the skin.

hypotension—low blood pressure.

hypothalamus (hye-poh-THAL-ah-mus)—located just above the brain stem, it is about the size of an almond and is responsible for certain types of metabolism; also acts as a link between the endocrine and nervous systems.

hypothyroidism—condition characterized by deficient release of thyroid hormones.

hypovolemia (hye-poh-voh-LEE-mee-uh)—abnormally low blood volume in the body.

hypoxia—deficiency in the oxygen levels or the blood's ability to transport oxygen, wherein toxic levels of carbon dioxide are allowed to accumulate.

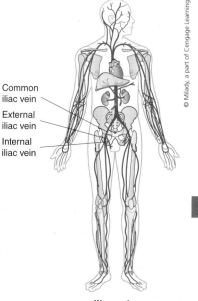

iliac (ILL-ee-ak) **veins**—veins found within the hips.

Imhotep—The world's first physician, who lived in Egypt and was the pharaoh's personal doctor around 2600 B.C.

imidazolidinyl urea (im-ih-DAZ-oh-lid-in-ul yoo-REE-uh)—antimicrobial agent, antibacterial preservative; very commonly used in cosmetics.

immunity—to have an immunologic resistance from disease by having been exposed to the antigen marker.

immunocompromised—referring to limited or reduced functioning of the immune system.

Common iliac vein
External iliac vein
Internal iliac vein

iliac veins

immunologic response—process by which the body reacts to a perceived threat and acts to eliminate it or neutralize it.

immunology—the study of the body defenses against disease.

impedance—resistance or obstruction of electrical flow. Commonly occurs when radiofrequency energy comes in contact with tissue.

impetigo (im-peh-TYE-goh)—skin infection from staphylococcal or streptococcal bacteria; often seen in children.

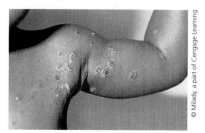

impetigo

173

inactive ingredient—ingredients that do not function actively; fragrances or carriers.

incretin mimetic (in-KREE-tin mih-MET-ik) **agent**—a class of drug which tricks the body into producing insulin as a means of treating type II diabetes.

indications—any sign or circumstance that a particular treatment is appropriate or warranted.

inert—will not react with other substances.

infarct—an area of tissue that becomes necrotic due to failure of the blood supply to deliver oxygen.

infected—contaminated with tissue-damaging microorganisms.

inferior—lower than.

inflamammary incision—for breast augmentation surgery, when the incision is made under the fold of the breast.

inflammatory bone disorders—generic term for any disease which results in bone inflammation, such as SAPHO.

inflammatory phase—early wound healing phase during which blood and fluid collect and substances begin to fight infection and promote healing.

infrared—electromagnetic radiation found in the invisible spectrum of light from 755 to 1200 nm.

ingredient list—the list of product composition by weight on cosmetics and skin care products.

inhibin (in-HIB-in)—hormone that inhibits the follicle stimulating hormone (FSH). This hormone is responsible for the growth and development of the reproductive systems.

inner frontalis—the medial part of the frontalis muscle. Its contraction raises the brow and eyebrows, forming wrinkles in the forehead and creating a slant up toward the center in the eyebrows.

innervates—the supplying of muscles or other tissues with sensory or motor nerves.

innocuous—non-contaminated or nonthreatening.

inorganic pigments—man-made dyes common in applied cosmetics. Derived most commonly from iron oxides or blended with other oxidized minerals like titanium dioxide. Color range is wide. They are stable and nontoxic.

in-phase—a property of light waves traveling parallel and in the same direction.

insertion—point of attachment to the bone, where a given muscle ends.

insulator—a material or device that prevents or reduces the passage of heat or electricity.

insulin—essential hormone needed for the normal metabolic breakdown of glucose in the body.

insulin-dependent diabetes mellitus (IDDM)—*see* type 1 diabetes.

insult—an injury or a trauma which causes an inconsistency in tissue.

integumentary system (integument)—the skin and its appendages (nails, hair, and sweat and oil glands).

intense pulsed light (IPL)—A polychromatic, non-coherent, dispersive band of light commonly utilizing wavelengths from 500 to 1200 nm and a variety of filters to diminish areas of color, both red and brown, on skin (also called Foto Facial® or Photo Facial®).

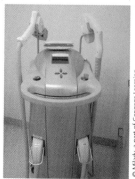

intense pulsed light

intercostal muscles—short muscles which fill in the gaps between the ribs, aiding respiration.

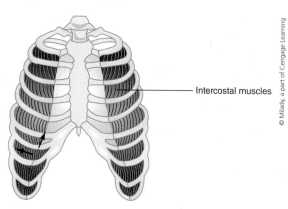

Intercostal muscles

internal obliques—inner layer of muscles which line the abdomen.

internal root sheath—the innermost layer of the hair follicle, closest to the hair.

interstitial (in-ter-STISH-ul) **tissue**—specialized absorbent tissue which lines the spaces between tissues or organs.

intestinal malabsorption—the inability of the intestines to effectively absorb nutrients from food, often resulting in malnutrition.

intracutaneous—within the skin.

intraoperatively—while in surgery.

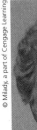
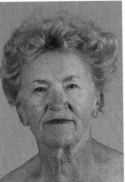

intrinsic aging—changes which would occur over time without the effects of any environmental factors.

in-vitro—in glass; an experiment in the laboratory.

in-vivo—any experiment conducted on a living subject.

involuntarily—acting without thought, by way of unconscious mechanisms, or by instinct.

iron oxide—a pigment for cosmetics.

irritable bowel syndrome—condition characterized by disturbances of normal bowel function of unknown etiology.

intrinsic aging

irritant—any agent that reacts on the skin, creating inflammation.

ischemia (iss-KEE-mee-ah)—a localized restriction of blood flow usually caused by an obstruction of normal circulation.

islets of Langerhans (LANG-er-hons)—clusters of cells in the pancreas that are responsible for the production of insulin.

isocetyl stearate (eye-soh-SEE-tel STEE-uh-rayt)—an emollient in cosmetic preparations.

isodecyl oleate (eye-soh-SEE-tel OH-lee-ayt)—emollient and wetting agent; also binds pigment.

isoluitane—a propellant used in aerosol products.

isopropyl alcohol—a colorless, flammable alcohol often used as a solvent.

isopropyl palmitate—from coconut oil; an emollient and moisturizer.

isotretinoin (eye-soh-trih-TIN-oyn)—*see* Accutane.

© Milady, a part of Cengage Learning

I

Japanese stone therapy—the therapeutic application of stones and massage with a facial or body treatment.

jaundice—symptom which is characterized by yellowing of the skin. Usually the result of improper liver functioning.

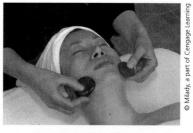

Japanese stone therapy

Jenner, Edward—British physician who discovered the vaccine for smallpox.

Jessner's solution—peel solution for the skin which is 14% resorcinol, 14% salicylic acid, 14% lactic acid in ethanol.

joules (JOOLS)—a measurement of a unit of energy from a pulsed laser or light source. One joule equals one watt per second.

Juvederm—trade name for popular hyaluronic acid dermal filler.

J

kakua (kuh-KOO-uh)—a nut from which darker-shaded dyes are made. Used in many cosmetic preparations.

kaolin (KAY-oh-lin)—common aluminum silicate; used in masks, powders.

Kaposi's (KAP-oh-seez) **sarcoma**—a skin disorder characterized by multiple areas of cell proliferation which eventually become cancerous. Common in individuals with compromised immune systems, as is the case with HIV/AIDS.

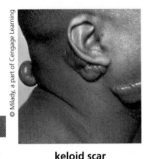

keloid scar

© Milady, a part of Cengage Learning

keloid (KEE-loyd) **scar**—scar formation in which tissue response is excessive in relation to normal tissue repair.

keratin (KER-uh-tin)—a protein found in the skin, hair, and nails that helps guard against bacterial or viral invasion. It is insoluble in water, weak acids, or alkalis.

keratinization—a progressive maturation to the keratinocyte and its movement through the epidermis to the stratum corneum. The keratinocyte eventually dies as it reaches the skin surface. The regular exfoliation of the dead skin cells results in a healthier skin appearance. Many aesthetic treatments are geared toward accomplishing as much.

keratinocytes—the primary cell in the skin, hair, or nails that produces keratin.

keratolysis—separation of the skin cells in the epidermis.

keratolytic—an agent that causes the keratinocytes to separate and ultimately leads to their destruction.

keratoses (ker-uh-TOH-sis)—any condition of the skin characterized by excessive horny growth.

keratotic plugs—loose keratin debris which clogs pores in acne.

ketoacidosis—abnormally high levels of ketone bodies; a compound which is a byproduct of fat metabolism.

kg—kilogram, a unit of weight measurement.

khite—Arabic word for threading technique for hair removal.

kinetin—type of cytokinin which aids cell division.

Kneipp (NIPE) **body wraps**—therapeutic body treatment which envelops a body part with wet and dry, hot and cold cloths that are applied for specific times. Developed in the nineteenth century by a German priest named Sebastian Kneipp.

KOH—potassium hydroxide/caustic potash/potassium lye.

kojic (KOH-jik) **acid**—skin-bleaching agent derived from bacteria of a Japanese mushroom. Used to treat a variety of skin dyschromias.

kola (KOH-luh) **nut**—African nut tree commonly used for strong stimulant qualities, as it contains high levels of caffeine. Medicinally, it is used as an herbal bronchodialator.

K

L—liter; basic metric unit of fluid measurement.

lacrimal (LAK-rih-mal)—pertaining to the tear ducts.

lactic acid—alpha-hydroxy acid originally derived from milk that is now produced synthetically. It is used in skin care products as an emollient, moisturizer, and preservative. Also used as a peeling agent.

lactogenic hormone—a hormone that induces the secretion of milk; prolactin.

lamellar granules—lipid-rich organelles that assist in producing the Natural Moisturizing Factor (NMF).

lamellar ichthyosis—a rare inherited disease associated with dry skin due to lamellar desquamation. Shows up soon after birth. The symptoms include scaling of the skin which is caused by an increase in the production of keratinocytes. In adulthood, the areas of the disease change and are more commonly found in the joints where the skin rubs together.

laneth-10—for emulsifying lanolin in cosmetic preparations.

Langelier (LONZH-el-yay) **index**—also called the saturation index; is a chemical equation that is used to diagnose the water balance and includes testing the water for pH, temperature, calcium hardness, and total alkalinity. Water with a high rating on this scale is often referred to as "hard water" and is associated with drying and irritation of the skin.

Langerhans (LANG-er-hons)—Cells found in the skin involved with immunity.

lanolin alcohol—emollient and emulsifier used in water in oil systems. Thought to be an allergen, this is a controversial product; however, studies show low incidence of allergy or irritation.

lanugo (luh-NOO-goh)—soft, downy hair present on fetuses in utero and infants at birth.

lap band—type of bariatric surgery during which a band is inserted around the upper part of the stomach, limiting the amount of food intake.

lapsana (lap-SAH-nuh)—prolific herb with antioxidant properties. Used as a protective agent of the skin in cosmetic preparations.

larynx—the cartilage that houses the vocal cords.

L-Ascorbic Acid—*see* vitamin C.

LASER—a device that produces an intense, coherent, directional beam of light by stimulating electronic or molecular transitions. Acronym for Light Amplification by Stimulated Emission of Radiation. Used in a variety of esthetic treatments including hair removal and skin resurfacing. Different types of lasers are effective for different treatments.

laser treatment controlled area (LTCA)—the specific room in which a laser treatment is performed and specific regulations, policies, and procedures are enforced by law. In this space, only certain personnel and people are permitted while treatments are being performed, and certain safety precautions, such as eye protection, are enforced.

latent—a stage of development; present but not visible.

late onset acne—acne which occurs after adolescence.

lateral—located on the side.

latissimus dorsal—large flat muscles which span the back.

lauramide—stabilizes foam; builds viscosity.

laureth 1 to 23—contains emulsifying properties.

lauric acid—stabilizes foam.

lauroyl lysine—amino acid; used as a skin conditioner.

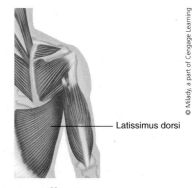

Latissimus dorsi

© Milady, a part of Cengage Learning

lauryl alcohol—skin conditioner; emollient.

lavandula angustifolia (lav-AN-doo-luh an-gus-tee-FOH-lee-uh) **(lavender essential oil)**—calming, healing; a good choice for sensitive skin.

lavender—primarily used as a fragrance and an aromatherapy calming agent; also thought to have antibacterial qualities in herbal preparations.

laxity—loose and without firmness; a phenomenon familiar to skin as it ages.

lecithin (LES-ih-thin)—emulsifier and antioxidant found in soybeans and eggs; for cosmetic use.

LED—*see* light-emitting diode.

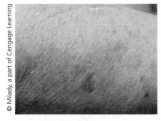

© Milady, a part of Cengage Learning

lentigines

Granulocytes

• Neutrophils

• Eosinophils

• Basophils

Agranulocytes

• Lymphocytes

• Monocytes

Leukocytes
(white blood cells, or WBCs)

© Milady, a part of Cengage Learning

lentigines (len-TIHJ-eh-neez)—flat brown spots appearing on aged or sun-exposed skin. Commonly called "sun spots" or by the misnomer "liver spots" although they are not related to any liver disease.

lesion—singular unusual or discontinuous spot on the skin. Isolated or in discontinuous clusters, there can be many etiologies, some more serious than others.

lethargy—feelings of excessive sluggishness or tiredness over an extended period of time.

leucocytes (LOO-koh-sites)—white blood cells or corpuscles.

leukemia—general term for any specific type of cancer affecting the blood-forming cells in the bone marrow, liver, spleen, and lymph nodes. Characterized by excessive and abnormal white blood cell proliferation.

leukocyte (LOO-koh-site)—white blood cells without granules with vital involvement in immune responses; they include the subsets lymphocytes and monocytes.

leukopenia—unusual deficiency in white blood cells. It may be temporary or long-term and indicative of a more serious condition.

leukotriene (loo-koh-TRY-een) **antagonist**—agent which acts as an inhibitor of leukotrienes, a chemical mediator of inflammation and usual suspect in the allergic response.

LEV—*see* local exhaust ventilators.

levator labii superioris (lih-VAY-ter LAY-bee-eye soo-peer-ee-OR-is)—muscle which lies below the nose to below the eyelids; acts to lift the lip.

Levulan—drug used for photodynamic treatment for certain skin conditions, such as acne or actinic keratosis. It acts to make certain cells more sensitive to light.

Leydig (LYE-dig) **cells—** also called interstitial cells of Leydig, located adjacent to the seminiferous tubules in the testicle. They secrete testosterone.

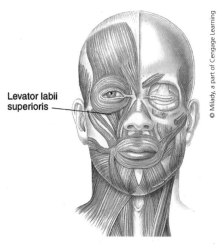

Levator labii superioris

LGAC—*see* laser-generated air contaminants.

libido—pertaining to sexual desire. May be compromised or exaggerated by certain medications, specifically those which affect the adrenal gland.

lichenification (lye-ken-if-ih-KAY-shun)—hardening and thickening of the skin as a result of repetitive irritation or physical manipulation.

lichen (LYE-ken) **simplex chronicus—**thickening of the skin in a specific area as a result of physical manipulation, such as might occur from scratching or rubbing in excess over a period of time.

licorice—dried root that contains glycyrrhetic acid; used as an anti-inflammatory and a flavoring agent in some cosmetic preparations.

lidocaine (LYE-doh-kayn)—common drug used for local anesthetic, meaning it does not cause total sensory deprivation, only sensory deprivation in the area it is topically applied or injected.

ligation—the act of tying a duct or blood vessel; to close off.

ligature—a tying or binding mechanism; suture or other device.

light-emitting diode (LED)—a device that is made up of panels of tiny diodes that are pulsed at an exclusive array sequence to trigger a photo-biochemical response.

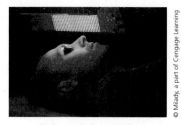

light emitting diode

linear—arranged in the form of a line.

lingual—pertaining to the tongue.

lining—(1) a permanent makeup technique for lip liner and eye liner (2) to be inside a perimeter.

linoleic (lih-NOH-lee-ik) **acid**—emulsifier, improves dry skin; also known as Omega 6. Common in many cosmetic preparations.

linoleic (lih-NOH-lee-ik) **acid triglyceride**—emollient that penetrates the skin well but is unstable and subject to rapid spoilage when used in cosmetic preparations.

lipase (LYE-pays)—sugar produced by the liver or pancreas that is responsible for the breakdown and digestion of ingestible fats.

lipid—fat or fat-like substances (descriptive, not chemical). Any substance with a high degree of viscosity as well as lubricative qualities: fatty or oily. Usually refers to biologic functions.

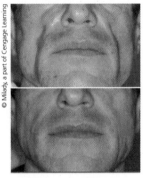

lipodystrophy—abnormal disruption in lipids as a result of compromised adipose tissues.

lipoprotein—the bond of a simple protein and a lipid; cholesterol.

liposome—sac formed when particular lipids are added to a water-based delivery solution, creating a seal that encapsulates the solution. They can be used to slowly release a drug into the body.

liposuction—removal of fat through surgical means.

lipodystrophy

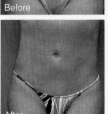

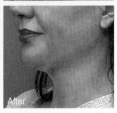

liposuction

LipoThene gel—jelly-like cosmetic emollient.

local exhaust ventilators (LEV)—smoke evacuator used in esthetic environments.

long QT syndrome—rare inborn heart condition contracted in utero. Can result in palpitations, irregular heartbeats, and even sudden death.

© Milady, a part of Cengage Learning

LTCA—*see* laser treatment controlled area.

lumen—the inside cavity or passage of a tubular structure such as a vein.

lupus—general term for a recurring, progressive, multisymptom autoimmune disease with unknown etiology; has many subcategories which are not limited to the skin. Can be systemic.

luteinizing (LOO-tee-eh-nye-zing) **hormone**—hormone which stimulates the corpus luteum, it also exhibits primary sexual characteristics in both males and females.

lymph—a colorless fluid that is involved in immune defenses and that removes foreign matter and cell debris.

lymphatic drainage—technique of manually or mechanically flushing sluggish lymphatic vessels and glands.

lymphatic vessels—tubes through which lymph flows through its network (*see* illustration on next page).

lymphedema (lim-feh-DEE-muh)—abnormal swelling of a limb due to impairment or excessive production in the flow of the lymph glands due to surgery and/or radiation therapy. Seen commonly in post-mastectomy patients.

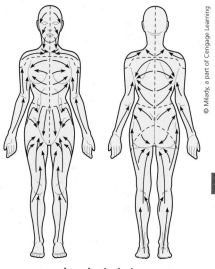

lymphatic drainage

© Milady, a part of Cengage Learning

lymph nodes—small glands which store the wastes collected by lymphocytes (*see* illustration on next page).

lymphocyte (LIM-foh-site)—white blood cells involved in the body's immune system; their numbers increase in the presence of infection.

lysine (LYE-seen)—amino acid for skin conditioning.

lysis—to dissolve or break apart.

lysogenic stage—cycle of viral activity during which the virus has attached to the cell and lies dormant.

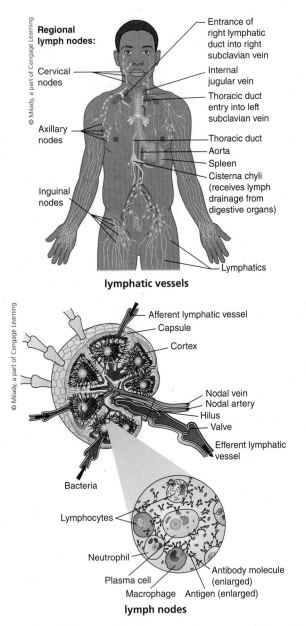

© Milady, a part of Cengage Learning

Regional lymph nodes:

Cervical nodes

Axillary nodes

Inguinal nodes

Entrance of right lymphatic duct into right subclavian vein

Internal jugular vein

Thoracic duct entry into left subclavian vein

Thoracic duct

Aorta

Spleen

Cisterna chyli (receives lymph drainage from digestive organs)

Lymphatics

lymphatic vessels

© Milady, a part of Cengage Learning

Afferent lymphatic vessel

Capsule

Cortex

Nodal vein

Nodal artery

Hilus

Valve

Efferent lymphatic vessel

Bacteria

Lymphocytes

Neutrophil

Plasma cell

Macrophage

Antibody molecule (enlarged)

Antigen (enlarged)

lymph nodes

lysosome—a cell organelle that contains water-destroying enzymes that help digest proteins and carbohydrates dividing them into components which are necessary and unnecessary to optimal bodily function.

macrophages (MAK-roh-fayjs)—primary phagocytic cells of the immune system in the skin; scavengers that clear debris in tissue injury.

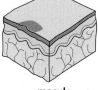

Localized changes in skin color of less than 1 cm in diameter
Example: Freckle

© Milady, a part of Cengage Learning

macule

macule (MAK-yool)—flat area of altered color or texture, less than one cm, not associated with texture changes.

maculopapular—eruptions of both macules and papules.

magnesium—common mineral found throughout the body and in nature. In the body, it activates enzymes necessary to amino acid/protein synthesis, helps regulate body temperature, and contributes to neuromuscular activity.

magnesium aluminium silicate—thickener used in cosmetic preparations.

magnesium ascorbyl (as-KOR-bil) **phosphate**—water-soluble whitening agent which is a form of ascorbic acid.

magnetic resonance imaging (MRI)—Noninvasive diagnostic technique that produces computerized images of internal body tissues and is based on nuclear magnetic resonance of atoms within the body that are induced by the application of radio waves. It is most often used to diagnose conditions affecting internal body tissues such as muscles or kidneys.

magnifying lamp—an illuminated lamp combined with magnification lenses that magnify the client's skin, assisting the esthetician in the analysis component of the facial treatment.

major depression—most severe type of depression,

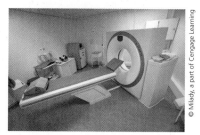

© Milady, a part of Cengage Learning

magnetic resonance imaging

characterized by severe and frequent instances of low mood, loss of interest, loss of energy, weight changes, changes in appetite, changes in sleep patterns, fatigue, inability to concentrate, feelings of low self-worth, and possibly thoughts of suicide.

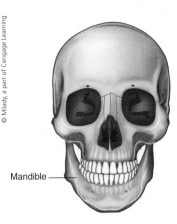

© Milady, a part of Cengage Learning

Malar prominence

malar (MAY-ler)—relating to the mala, or the cheek.

malar (MAY-ler) **prominence**—projection of the cheek bone.

malic (MAL-ik) **acid**—alpha-hydroxy acid originally derived from apples; now prepared synthetically. Used therapeutically in the treatment of fine lines associated with aging.

malignant—cancerous, or harmful to one's health.

malnutrition—any condition which causes a lack of nutritional substances for the body to use and distribute.

malpighian (mal-PIG-ee-un) **layer**—a skin layer made of the stratum mucosum and the stratum germinativum.

malpositioned—in the wrong position.

© Milady, a part of Cengage Learning

Mandible

mammoplasty—plastic or cosmetic surgery of the breast.

mandible—the lower jawbone.

mandibular—pertaining to the mandible.

manual tap—non-motorized method of implanting color into the skin during permanent makeup procedures.

MAOIs—*see* monoamine oxidase inhibitors.

margin—(1) a line (2) in anatomy, the edges of a structure.

margination—neither sharp nor defined.

masks—(1) esthetic treatments which contain active ingredients in high concentrations intended to intensify the treatment and work on the principles of occlusion. There are many different types of masks and also an equally diverse amount of conditions for which they are used. Generally speaking, masks are a milder treatment in the medical spa environment, often used as a relaxing adjunct therapy to more aggressive therapies such as a peel or an injectable treatment. (2) facial coverings used by physicians and other personnel as a universal protection of the nose and mouth.

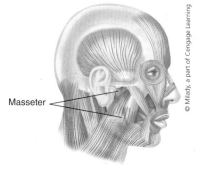

© Milady, a part of Cengage Learning

masseter (mah-SEE-ter)—muscle that closes the mouth; used for chewing.

Masseter

mast cells—large white blood cells present in the skin and other tissue which produce histamine and other acute symptoms of allergic reactions, such as anaphylaxis.

mastectomy—surgical removal of a breast.

mastication—to chew.

mastopexy (MAS-tuh-pek-see)—technical term for a breast lift.

material safety data sheet (MSDS)—document which contains vital data regarding the dispersal, properties, and effects of certain substances regulated by law.

M

maxilla—the upper jaw.

maximum permissible exposure (MPE)—the level of laser radiation to which the unexposed human eye can be exposed without hazardous tissue effects resulting in measurable damage.

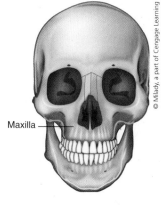

© Milady, a part of Cengage Learning

medial—in the middle.

medial thigh lift—type of body-contouring surgery by which excessive skin in the middle inner thigh is removed for patients who have undergone massive weight loss.

Maxilla

medicated products—products with ingredients to soothe or relax, but not necessarily cure a condition or symptom.

medispa—the fusion of medical services and spa services, found in a medical setting.

medulla (meh-DUL-uh)—the innermost layer of hair; composed of round cells; often absent in fine hair.

meglitinides (meg-LIT-in-ides)—class of drugs used in the treatment of type 2 diabetes which acts to increase insulin production in the pancreas.

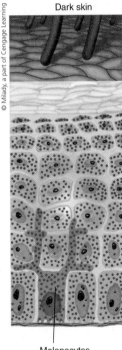

Dark skin

Melanocytes

melanocyte

Meissner's (MY-snerz) **corpuscles**—nerve endings in the skin that are sensitive to touch; found in the dermal papillae.

melaleuca alternifolia (mel-uh-LOO-kah altern-ee-FOH-lee-uh)—tea tree essential oil; popular for use as an antiseptic.

melanin—tyrosine-based amino acid that acts as a pigment in plants and animals. In humans, it is responsible for the color of skin, eyes, and hair. One of its primary functions is to act as a protectant from damaging effects of ultraviolet light.

melanocyte—type of cell found in the basal layer of the epidermis which produces melanin. Those with darker skin do not have more melanin, just more active cells.

melanogenisis—the process by which melanocytes produce melanin, and hence, skin pigment.

melanoma—a malignant, darkly pigmented mole or tumor of the skin.

Melaquin—3 percent concentration of hydroquinone. Brand name for a skin lightening medication used to treat dyschromias.

melasma—A chronic hyperpigmentation skin disorder that can be a result of prolonged unprotected sun exposure, birth control pills, hormone replacement therapy, and pregnancy. Caused from an overproduction

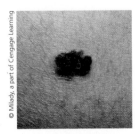

melanoma

M

of melanin. Presents as reddish-brown blotchy spots or areas on the face or other parts of the skin. Also called cholasma.

melasma gravidarum—commonly called "mask of pregnancy"; brown spots of the face resulting from an overproduction of melanin.

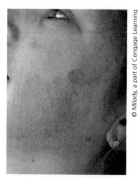

melatonin—produced in the pineal gland; responsible for the sleep patterns in human beings.

melting points—temperature at which a solid begins to liquefy.

membrane—thin barrier.

menopause—point in a woman's aging when ovulation and menstruation cease. While it is associated with

melasma gravidarum

many hormonal and physical changes, effects on the skin include drying and loss of elasticity.

mental illness—umbrella term for any condition which results in a measurable dysfunction of mental or psychotic functioning.

mentum—the chin.

Merkel cells—usually close to nerve endings and may be involved in sensory perception.

metabolic alkalosis—increased alkalinity in the body resulting from decreased acids.

M

metabolism—physical and chemical reactions in the cell which sustain life, particularly the ongoing conversion of food into energy and the distribution of required biochemicals throughout the body. An individual's metabolism will vary greatly from one person to the next, resulting in a great amount of variation in appearance, weight, and overall health.

metastable—in an apparent state of equilibrium, but likely to change to a more truly stable state if conditions change. For example, a condition's symptoms may be made metastable by treating the symptoms, whereas

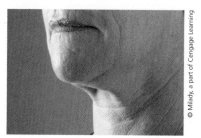

mentum

true stability could be achieved by treating the condition itself.

metastasis—the spread of a cancer.

metatastic—pertaining to the act of movement of malignant cells from one part of the body to another; *see* metastasis.

methicillin-resistant staphylococcus aureus—also known as MRSA or MERSA, it is a serious, potentially deadly, antibiotic-resistant strain of the staphylococcus bacterium. Presents similar to a painful boil on the skin. Commonly found in pools, hot tubs, locker rooms, or other heated and moist environments hospitable to bacteria growth. Also found on the hands and in the nasal passages of hospital workers; commonly found in hospital or nursing home settings.

methicone—silicone used in cosmetic powders.

mica—fine mineral powder comprising silicates and metals that is commonly used as glitter in cosmetic preparations.

microgenia—small chin.

micrometer—a unit of length equal to a millionth of a meter, or a micron.

microthermal zones (MTZ)—as in a column of tissue heated up by the laser system.

mid-facelift—plastic surgery intended to remove wrinkling and excess skin from the lower eyelid to the jawline.

M

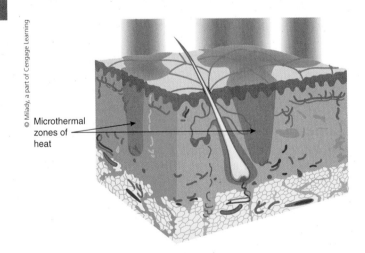

© Milady, a part of Cengage Learning

Microthermal zones of heat

migration—(1) pertaining to esthetics, the movement within the skin so that it is visible beyond the desired location of implantation (2) to move.

milia (mil-ee-uh)—plugs caused by obstruction of sebaceous matter; closed comedo.

miliaria (mil-ee-AYR-ee-uh)—commonly referred to as prickly heat; a skin condition characterized by isolated patches of itchy bumps.

milliamperemeter—a device that measures electric current in units of 1/1000 of an ampere.

milliamperes—units of electric current, one of which equals 1/1000 of an ampere.

milliequivalent—a chemical equivalent; one one-thousandth.

mineralocorticoids—hormone responsible for fluid balance.

mineral oil—natural oil good in cleansers; however, comedogenicity depends on the level of product refinement.

mitosis—the process by which a cell divides into two daughter cells (*see* Figure 2.2 on page 11).

mL—milliliter; unit of liquid measurement.

moderate-depth peels—peels in which the depth extends into the papillary dermis.

modify—to qualify or limit the meaning of an object.

modulate—the ability to stimulate, regulate, or change the cellular function or its intended result.

moisturizer—any ingredient or preparation that replaces or protects the loss of moisture; a combination of a humectant and an emollient with lipid replacement qualities intended to prevent skin from drying out. In doing so, it is a vital component of a client's daily skin care regimen.

molds—growth of certain fungi on a host surface.

molecular weight—average weight of an element, molecule, or compound.

monoamine oxidase inhibitors (MAOIs)—a class of drugs used in treatment for depression. The exact mode of their action is not quite understood.

monochromatic—light consisting of one wavelength of the color spectrum of light.

monocytes—large phagocytic white blood cells which roam the bloodstream, neutralizing pathogens.

monosaccharides (mon-oh-SAK-uh-rides)—simple sugar; carbohydrates' building blocks.

moor mud—a natural peat preparation, rich in organic matter, proteins, vitamins, and trace minerals able to penetrate the skin, influencing enzymatic and hormone activity.

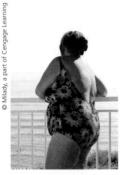

morbid obesity—excessive and unhealthy weight in adults with a body mass index greater than or equal to 30. Individuals who are considered morbidly obese have higher instances of heart disease, diabetes, and other conditions which are considered dangerous to one's well-being.

morbilliform—a rash resembling measles.

motor neuropathic diseases—any disorder which causes reduced-capacity muscle use or complete paralysis on one or more areas.

morbid obesity

mottling—skin condition characterized by patchy discoloration of the skin; red or brown.

MPE—*see* maximum permissible exposure.

MRI—*see* magnetic resonance imaging.

MRSA—*see* methicillin-resistant staphylococcus aureus.

MSDS—*see* material safety data sheet.

MTZ—*see* microthermal zones.

mucocutaneous toxicity—poisoning of the skin and mucous membranes.

mucopolysaccharides (myoo-koh-pol-ee-SAK-uh-rides)—sugars and proteins with the ability to bind to water. They also form the ground substance in cells. With regard to skin moisture, they reduce TEWL.

mucositis (myoo-koh-SYE-tis)—inflammation of the mucous membranes.

mucosocutaneous (myoo-koh-soh-kyoo-TAY-nee-us)—pertaining to the mucous membranes and skin.

mucous membranes—tissue linings in internal tracts which require lubrication, secrete mucus, and communicate with air.

mud—used in esthetic treatments to refine, exfoliate, or add nutrients to the skin.

mulberry root—botanical used in cosmetic and esthetic preparations for treatment of dyschromias.

multiple myeloma (my-eh-LOH-mah)—malignant proliferation of plasma cells resulting in a tumor; condition characterized by tumor cells infiltrating the bone and bone marrow.

multiplex technology—the emission of two separate wavelengths of laser light from one device.

muscle fibers—cylindrical, multinucleated cells which can expand and contract voluntarily or involuntarily.

muscular system—complex network of tissue which supports, moves, and postures the body.

musculature—pertaining to a system or arrangement of muscle tissue.

musculocutaneous—pertaining to muscle and skin.

muslin strips—thin, plain-weave cotton cloth used for removing wax from the skin during wax hair-removal treatments.

myalgia (my-AL-jee-ah)—either symptomatic or asymptomatic muscle pain.

mycosis fungoides (my-KOH-sis FUN-goyds)—a rare T-cell skin cancer, non-Hodgkins T-cell lymphoma, which has skin manifestations on the scalp and trunk that itch.

myelogenous (my-eh-LOH-jen-us)—originating in the bone marrow.

myocardial ischemia (my-oh-KAR-dee-al iss-KEE-mee-ah)—temporary restriction in normal blood flow to the heart and cardiac muscles.

M

myocardium (my-oh-KAR-dee-um)—striated muscular tissue within the heart which facilitates the propulsion of the blood between chambers.

myofilaments—tiny tubules which make up the muscle tissue.

myristic (muh-RIS-tik) **acid**—cleansing agent that works especially well when combined with potassium.

myristyl (muh-RIS-til) **alcohol**—emollient; used in hand creams and other esthetic preparations.

myxedema (mik-seh-DEE-mah)—metabolic and skin condition characterized by overfunctioning of the thyroid gland (hyperthyroidism). Presents with mental and physical impairment.

N

nanometer—metric measurement indicating a billionth of a meter.

narcotic—term for any drug that is both physically and psychologically addictive but has medicinal benefits, most often pain management from opiates.

nare (NAYR)—a nostril.

NASHA—*see* non-animal stabilized hyaluronic acid.

nasolabial—pertaining to the nose and mouth.

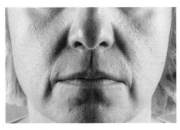

nasolabial folds

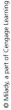

nasolabial folds—wrinkling associated with the lines that connect the nose to the lip; commonly called smile lines or "parentheses" of the face.

nasopharyngitis (nay-zoh-far-in-JYE-tis)—inflammation of the nose and throat.

nasopharynx (nay-zoh-FAR-inks)—point where the nasal passage intersects with the throat.

natural—"from nature"; describes subjectively the idea that the products are not synthetic but come from nature. Cosmetically speaking, it is not a dependable or legal term and should not be the only qualifier for selection of a product.

natural color—pertaining to unprocessed cosmetic dyes with earthen origins; less toxic but more likely to fade or wash away.

natural moisturizing factor (NMF)—compound found only in top layer of skin that gives cells their ability to bind with water, moisturizing the skin. The inability of these compounds to function or an imbalance in these compounds results in drier skin and the appearance of premature aging. As one ages, there is a tendency to age more quickly as these compounds become less abundant.

necrosis—death of cells, when tissue is deprived of blood supply.

neonatal acne—type of acne affecting newborn babies.

neonatal cephalic pustulosis (nee-oh-NAY-tuhl suh-FAL-ik pus-tyoo-LOH-sis)—form of neonatal acne.

nephropathy (neh-FROP-ah-thee)—kidney disease accompanied by inflammation and degenerative, sclerotic lesions of the kidney.

nephrotoxicity—kidney toxicity.

neuroblastoma—a certain type of malignant tumor originating in nerve tissue of the brain and spinal cord.

neurocutaneous—pertaining to the nerves and the skin.

neurogenic bladder—improper bladder functioning resulting in overactivity or underactivity of normal urinary function associated with the central nervous system and peripheral nerves involved in urination.

neurohypophysis (new-roh-hye-POF-is-is)—hormone-secreting part of the pituitary gland; posterior portion.

neuroleptic drugs—any medication that changes normal brain patterns and, thus, behavior, resulting in physical and mental impairment. Often have a calming or sedative result. Used to treat psychotic conditions.

neuromuscular junction—anatomical point where muscles interpret nerve impulses into voluntary muscle movement.

neuromuscular junctional disorders—any disorder which affects the neuromuscular junction.

neurons (NEW-ronz)—nervous system cells which process and transmit nerve impulses.

neuropathy—disease of the nerves or nervous system.

neurotransmitter—substances that travel across synapses to act on a target cell. Critical component to dynamic muscle movement and proper brain activity.

neutral—any agent which has a pH that is exactly 7.0. Neither acidic nor alkaline.

neutralization—process by which active agents lose their potency, either with the addition of another agent, or the loss of time.

neutropenia—abnormally low levels of neutrophil cells in the body.

neutrophil (NEW-troh-fil)—most common type of phagocytic white blood cells that kill bacteria by traveling to a wound site and digesting bacteria.

neutrophilic dermatosis (new-troh-FIL-ik der-muh-TOH-sis)—aka Sweet's syndrome, papules and nodules which combine to form plaques. Usually occurs on the face and neck.

N

niacin (NYE-uh-sin)—also called vitamin B3. Commonly found in yeast, meat, and as an additive to esthetic preparations. Aids in hormone production, DNA, and wound healing; important for metabolism.

niacinamide (nye-uh-SIN-uh-mide)—vitamin B. Common in meats, grains, fish, and eggs. Has been shown to decrease transepidermal water loss (TEWL), but can be toxic in high quantities.

nicotinic (nik-oh-TIN-ik) **acid**—*see* niacin.

Nikolsky's (nih-KOHL-skeez) **sign**—an autoimmune condition of the skin characterized by blistering or epidermal separation upon manipulation.

nipple-areolar complex—pertaining to the nipple and the areola.

NMF—*see* natural moisturizing factor.

nocturia (nok-TOO-ree-uh)—excessive and frequent urination at night.

nodule—elevated solid lesion greater than 1 cm.

nodulocystic (nod-jeh-leh-SIS-tik)—pertaining to nodules and cysts.

nodulocystic (nod-jeh-leh-SIS-tik) **acne**—severe acne which presents with nodules and cysts.

non-animal stabilized hyaluronic (HYE-eh-loo-ron-ik) **acid**—refined heterologous hyaluronic acids, for instance, Restylane.

non-Hodgkin's lymphoma—a certain type of malignant cancer originating in the lymphatic system.

non-immunogenic—unlikely to cause a hypersensitive or antigenic reaction.

non-inflammatory—pertaining to a skin condition or agent which is not accompanied by inflammation.

non-insulin-dependent diabetes mellitus—*see* type 2 diabetes.

nonionic surfactant—agent without electrical charge.

nonsteroidal anti-inflammatory drugs (NSAIDS)—class of drugs that includes ibuprofen; used to treat pain and inflammation.

nonsurgical esthetic skin care—Any noninvasive procedure, performed by an esthetician or registered nurse, that is intended to improve overall skin health and appearance. Not to be confused with lack of pain or downtime, as both are significantly less. However, the potential for pain and proper healing exist in these less aggressive skin care treatments as well.

nontransient erythema (ayr-ih-THEE-muh)—rosacea which presents with papules and pustules.

norepinephrine (nor-ep-ih-NEF-rin)—hormone produced in the adrenal medulla which acts as a vasoconstrictor.

normal saline—water combined with pH-balanced sodium solution, used to mix injectables or irrigate wounds.

normal sinus rhythm—an electrical impulse which regulates the normal heartbeat, usually at a pace of 60 to 100 beats per minute as measured by an electrocardiogram.

Novocain—a trademarked name for a synthetic anesthetic drug most commonly used intravenously for oral or dental procedures.

NPO—from the Latin non per os, meaning not by mouth; medical shorthand meaning nothing to eat or drink .

nucleic acid—basic nucleotide subunits; part of DNA structure.

nucleus—considered the "brain of the cell," organelle which contains genetic material and manages the functions of an individual cell.

nymphaea alba (NIM-fee-uh AL-buh) **(water lily extract)**— soothing and calming for the skin.

nystagmus (nis-TAG-mus)—involuntary and constant movement of the eyeball.

N

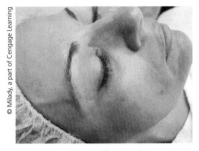

Obagi Blue Peel

Obagi (oh-BOZH-ee) **Blue Peel**—simplified, uniform, user-friendly professional-strength TCA peel solution indicated for all skin types. Created by Dr. Zein Obagi.

oblique (oh-BLEEK)—(1) muscle used to twist the torso (2) slanting or inclined; 45-degree angle.

Obsessive-Compulsive Disorder (OCD)—anxiety disorder characterized by perpetual and excessive thoughts and activities which interfere with the normal functioning of the affected individual. Certain esthetic conditions such as trichotillimania and Body Dysmorphic Disorder are thought by some to be forms of OCD.

occlusion (uh-KLOO-zhun)—to close, obstruct, or grind together.

occlusive agent—(1) the process of closing or obstruction (2) a product that prevents the skin from losing moisture or reduces TEWL, for example, Vaseline.

occupational acne—generic term for any type of acne that is a result of oil and other chemicals present at the place of work or where an individual spends a great deal of time.

Occupational Safety and Hazard Administration (OSHA)—federal agency responsible for defining and regulating safety in the workplace. OSHA regulations must be adhered to at all times in the event of a workplace incident. Failure to comply can result in heavy fines and/or revocation of operational licensure.

octocrylene (ok-toh-KRIH-leen)—water-resistant sunscreen agent; UVB blocker.

octyl salicylate (OK-til sal-ih-SIL-ayt)—sunscreen; non-comedogenic.

oenothera biennis (ee-noh-THEE-ruh bye-EN-is)—evening primrose oil; used for dry skin.

off-label—use other than the stated purpose; not FDA approved for that use.

Ohm's law—the law of physics that states that electric current is directly proportional to the voltage applied to a conductor and inversely proportional to that conductor's resistance.

oil—viscous fluid. It is an emollient, a lubricant, and unable to bind with water in natural circumstances. Oils are commonly found in all plants and animals and, as extracts, are common ingredients in cosmetic, esthetic, and food recipes.

oil acne—type of occupational acne associated with oil or oily materials.

ointment base—inactive or inert ingredients added to a medicinal or therapeutic preparation.

Olea europaea (OH-lee-uh yoo-roh-PEE-uh)—olive oil; used as an emollient and lubricant in cosmetic preparations.

oleic (oh-LEE-ik) **acid**—non-edible Omega–9 oil derived from olives, used as an emollient; skin-penetrating properties in esthetic preparations and an excipient in pharmaceuticals.

oligoelement—a trace element.

oligohydrosis—condition characterized by excessively low water levels in the body and reduced capacity to perspire.

oligospermia (ol-ih-go-SPER-mee-uh)—low sperm count; temporary or permanent; primary or secondary condition.

oliguria (ol-ih-GOO-ree-uh)—decreased production of urine as a result of dehydration or other conditions.

onychomycosis (on-ih-koh-my-KOH-sis)—parasitic fungal infection of the nails.

opaque colors—non-transparent colors, impervious to light; have covering power.

ophthalmic—pertaining to the eye.

opportunistic mycoses—a fungal infection that preys on hosts with compromised immunities.

O

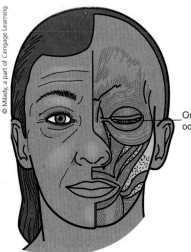

Orbicula oculi m.

optical cavity—the part of the laser that contains the active medium.

optical density (OD)—protection provided by a filter for a specific wavelength of light.

orbicularis oculi (or-bik-yeh-LAYR-is OK-yoo-lye)—muscle on the face that is responsible for opening and closing the eyelids.

organelles—micro-organs responsible for specific functions within a cell.

organic—(1) derived from living organisms (2) pertaining to organs (3) class of chemical compounds formed from carbon.

organism—a living thing.

orifice—aperture; hole opening into a body cavity.

origin—point where a given muscle begins; a beginning; point in time in which something begins; an individual's spiritual, physical, ethnic, or social history.

ornithine decarboxylase (OR-nih-theen dee-kar-BOK-suh-lays)—enzyme found in human skin which stimulates facial hair growth.

OSHA—*see* Occupational Safety and Health Administration.

osmosis—diffusion of a fluid through a semipermeable membrane; concentrations change when the solution moves through the membrane.

osmotic—pertaining to the ability of a substance to pass through a membrane that separates the substance from other materials.

osteitis (os-tee-EYE-tis)—inflammation of the bone.

osteoarthritis—joint condition characterized by chronic inflammation and degeneration of weight-bearing joints.

osteolytic (os-tee-oh-LIH-tik) **bone lesions**—condition characterized by inflammation and cysts on the bones.

otoplasty (OH-toh-plas-tee)—type of cosmetic surgery meant to remedy ears that stand out.

outer frontalis—the outer part of the frontalis muscle. Its contraction raises the lateral part of the brow and eyebrows, forming wrinkles in the lateral part of the forehead and an arched shape to the eyebrows (*see* illustration at bottom of page).

outer orbicularis oculi—eye muscle which acts to open and close the eyelids.

overactive bladder—condition characterized by abnormally high levels of bladder activity, resulting in frequent need to urinate.

over-the-counter (OTC)—any remedy which can be obtained without a doctor's prescription.

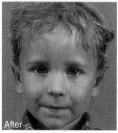

otoplasty

oxidation—a toxic reaction to prolonged exposure to oxygen.

oxygenate—to supply with oxygen.

oxyhemoglobin—oxygenated hemoglobin, a common chromophore found in the blood that is absorbed by certain visible wavelength(s) of light.

oxytocin (ok-sih-TOH-sin)—hormone which stimulates contractions of the womb during childbirth.

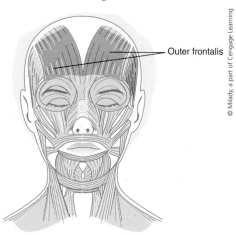

Outer frontalis

0

PABA—also known as para-aminobenzoic acid, it is the cousin of the B complex found in animals other than humans; PABA's most common use is that of an effective sunscreen; many people are allergic.

P. acnes bacteria—*see* propionibacterium.

Paget's (PAJ-its) **disease**—condition affecting the elderly characterized by inflammation of the bones.

palliative—a remedy that alleviates symptoms but does not cure the underlying condition.

palmar-plantar erythrodysesthesia (uh-rith-roh-dis-es-THEE-zhuh)—condition characterized by redness and pain on the palms and soles of the feet.

palpebra (PAL-puh-bruh)—eyelid; superior upper and inferior lower.

pancreas—vital hormone-producing organ of the abdominal region that is both exocrine and endocrine in nature.

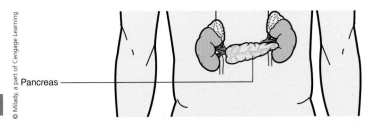

© Milady, a part of Cengage Learning

Pancreas

pancreatitis—condition characterized by inflammation of the pancreas.

pandemic—disease occurring over a wide geographic region.

panniculus—enormous amounts of loose skin around the midsection of individuals who have undergone massive weight loss.

panthenol (PAN-theh-nol)—vitamin B5, a moisturizer in esthetic preparations.

papain (puh-PAY-in)—papaya enzyme also found in pineapples, used as an exfoliant in esthetic preparations.

papillae (puh-PIL-ee)—cone-shaped elevation at the base of the bulb filled with the vascular component for the hair follicle.

papillary dermal wounding—any injury to the skin which reaches deep enough to cause bleeding.

papillary dermis—the most superficial layer of the dermis; housed between the basal layer of the epidermis and the reticular layer of the dermis (*see* Fig. 2–40 on page 56).

papillomatosis (pap-ih-LOH-muh-toh-sis)—condition characterized by widespread benign tumor growth.

papillomavirus (pap-ih-LOH-muh-vye-rus)—the virus with many subsets thought to be responsible for warts, cervical cancer, anal cancer, and other conditions.

papule (PAP-yool)—elevated solid lesion on the skin that is less than 1 cm.

Solid, elevated lesion less than 0.5 cm in diameter
Example: Warts, elevated nevi

© Milady, a part of Cengage Learning

papule

papulopustular (pap-yoo-loh-PUS-tyoo-lar) **eruptions**—lesions on the skin which present with both papules and pustules.

para-aminobenzoic acid—*see* PABA.

parabens (PAR-eh-bens)—most common preservatives in cosmetic products.

paradigm—a model or pattern which operates as a foundation for ideas, thoughts, or models expanded upon the original model or pattern.

parafango—a mixture of fango mud and paraffin used for therapeutic purposes in facials and body detox treatments.

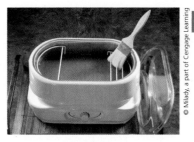

© Milady, a part of Cengage Learning

P

paraffin—a synthetic waxy crystalline agent obtained from distilled petroleum.

parahormone—a chemical substance produced from ordinary metabolism

parafango

which has a stimulating effect similar to that of a hormone, but doesn't originate from the endocrine system.

parasympathetic nervous system—targeted responses from certain organs of the body to respond to stimuli from the brain (for example, the narrowing of the pupil when the brain responds to brightening light).

parenteral—any drug delivery route other than oral; intramuscular, intravenous, subcutaneous.

paresthesia (par-es-THEE-zee-uh)—sensation of numbness and prickling resulting from restricted blood flow; often called "pins and needles."

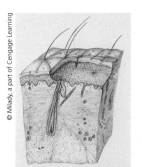

© Milady, a part of Cengage Learning

partial thickness wound

Parkinson's disease—progressive nervous system disease characterized by progressive tremors, muscular weakness, and rigidity.

Parsol 1789—preferred sunscreen ingredient that protects against photodamage and premature aging of the skin from exposure to UVA light.

partial thickness injury—a wound that penetrates only the epidermis or the upper layer of the papillary dermis. These wounds tend to heal quickly and without scarring. In more invasive esthetic treatments, such as laser or chemical, the ideal situation is to induce controlled partial thickness injuries to the skin.

Pasteur (pas-TYOOR), **Louis**—French scientist who discovered pasteurization.

patch—large macule on the skin greater than 2 cm; often the product of hypersensitivity or an allergic reaction.

patchouli (puh-CHOO-lee)—an essential oil derived from the leaves of the patchouli scrub.

patch test—to test a drug or treatment on a small patch of skin to determine the suitability of the product or treatment by the absence of allergic reaction.

pathogen—an agent, namely a bacteria or virus, capable of producing disease.

pathogenesis—the expected course of a disease or condition.

pathogenic bacteria—any bacteria which is responsible for disease or infection.

pathogenic fungi—any fungus which results in disease or infection.

P

pathology—the study of diseases and their courses in certain populations.

peat—an organic material produced as a heterogeneous mixture of natural materials in a rapid state of decomposition.

pectin—a thickener for cosmetics, jellies, and jams derived from citrus fruits.

pectoralis major—prominent muscles of the upper chest. Commonly referred to as the "pectorals" or "pecs." These muscles are responsible for pushing and pulling.

pedunculated (peh-DUN-kyoo-layt-ed)—having the qualities of a pendulum; having an attached part that dangles or oscillates.

peel depth—the degree to which a peeling agent penetrates.

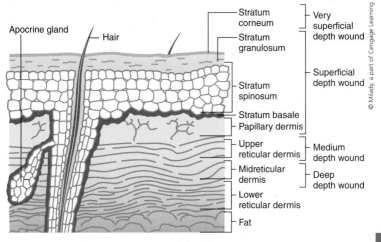

peel depth

peel percentage—related to peeling, it pertains to the solution mixture, not to be confused with pH. Typically, the higher the percentage the greater the amount of the active ingredient. .

pellon strips—a woven strip of soft paper used to remove hair and wax from the skin.

pentasodium pentate—emulsifier and agent for dissolving moisturizers.

peptic ulcer—a wearing down of normal tissue of the stomach and esophagus resulting in frequent stomach pain, especially after eating.

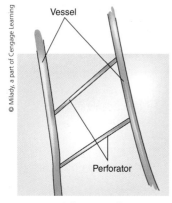

Vessel

Perforator

perforator veins

perforator veins—veins that connect deep veins and superficial veins.

periareolar (payr-ee-uh-REE-oh-lar) **incision**—during breast surgery, the incision made around the areola so as to eliminate or minimize scarring potential.

pericardial cavity—the space between the parietal pericardium and the epicardium; both contain lubricating fluids.

pericardium—the sac surrounding the heart (*see* Fig. 2–17 on page 29).

perifollicular edema (eh-DEE-muh)—irritation, erythema, and edema around the hair follicle seen frequently after a laser/light exposure.

perifolliculitis capitis abscedens et suffodiens (PCAS)—condition of the scalp of unknown etiology.

perimenopausal—time just before the cessation of menstruation and ovulation.

perimysium (payr-uh-MIZ-ee-um)—connective tissue which makes up muscle fiber bundles, which in turn make up muscle tissue.

perinasal—around the nose.

perineural—around a nerve.

periocular—around the eye.

perioral—around the mouth.

P

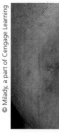

perioral dermatitis

perioral dermatitis—general term for the condition characterized by itching, redness, and irritation around the mouth.

periorbital—around the orbit of the eye.

periosteum (payr-ee-OS-tee-um)—fibrous material that covers the bones.

peripheral edema (eh-DEE-muh)—swelling resulting from fluid accumulation in the lower limbs, typically surrounding an injury point.

peripheral venous return—secondary system of blood return to the heart, in which muscles in the calves help push blood vertically against gravity.

permanent makeup—use of ink below the skin to replicate the effects of applied makeup for long-term esthetic purposes.

permeability—ability of a substance to allow another substance to pass through under pressure.

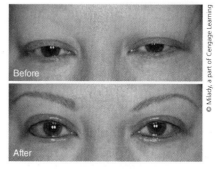

permanent makeup

permeate—reverse osmosis; to pass through.

persea gratissima (PER-see-uh grah-TIS-ih-muh)—also called avocado oil. Emollient; excellent for dry skin.

persistent acne—subset of acne vulgaris that begins in adolescence and continues into adulthood.

petit mal—a form of epileptic seizure marked by episodes of brief loss of consciousness without convulsions or falling. Sometimes referred to as a "staring spell."

petroleum jelly—a lubricant and emollient; an occlusive agent used for medical and esthetic purposes.

pH (potential of hydrogen)—the scale by which a material is characterized as being acidic (pH less than 7.0), alkaline (greater than 7.0), or neutral (7.0).

phagocytes (FAG-oh-sites)—waste-clearing white blood cells which consume bacteria. They are the first to arrive at potentially vulnerable entry points for opportunistic infections, hence being one of the body's very first lines of defense.

pharmaceutical—a drug or medicine to improve disease or illness that is regulated by governing agencies and usually prescribed by a physician.

pharynx (FAR-inks)—connects the mouth to the esophagus and the nasal cavity to the larynx.

phenol (FEE-nol) **(C₆H₅OH)**—also known as carbolic acid, a highly corrosive acid used in deep peel solutions, which dissolves cells in order to make room for newer and healthier ones; when used on the skin it will permanently depigment the skin, resulting in an inability to tan.

phenothiazines (fee-nuh-THYE-uh-zeens)—general name for a type of drug used to treat schizophrenic or psychotic disorders with a tranquilizing effect.

phenoxyethanol (fih-nok-see-ETH-eh-nol)—antimicrobial agent used with parabens in sunscreens.

phenyl dimethicone (FEN-nil dye-METH-ih-kohn)—inhibits foaming in esthetic preparations.

pheomelanin (fee-o-MEL-uh-nin)—the red to yellow tones of melanin apparent in skin and hair.

pheromone—a chemical substance, the release of which may affect the behavior or physiology of a recipient.

phlebitis (fleh-BYE-tis)—inflammation of the wall of a vein. Presents as a blotchy red, heated, and elevated area often near points of tissue injury. Individuals on certain types of medications are particularly prone to this condition.

phlebology (fleh-BOL-uh-jee)—that branch of anatomical science concerning veins and venous disease, particularly the safe withdrawal, storage, and testing of blood.

phobias—anxiety condition characterized by unwarranted fear such that it interferes with the normal functioning of the affected individual.

phoresis (foh-REE-sis)—the use of a galvanic current to force chemical solutions into unbroken skin.

phospholipids—contain phosphorus and fatty acids, the lipid components of the cell membrane.

phosphoric acid—used to adjust product pH in cosmetic preparations.

photoactive—capable of responding to light or light sources.

photodamage—damage caused by repeated and unprotected sun exposure over time; also called solar damage. It is well understood to be a major contributor to extrinsic aging. Appears as wrinkled skin, lentigines, and sometimes skin cancers—most especially basal cell carcinomas, also known as BCC.

photodynamic therapy—the use of a topical photosensitizing ALA (*see* Levulan) medication followed by irradiation with a visible light source to treat a variety of skin disorders, including acne.

photograph—necessary component of skin care treatment program which accurately documents the original skin condition, as to prove or disclaim treatment results. It is a vital component of the treatment as it can accurately prove results, or the lack thereof.

photomodulation—to use controlled light therapies to regulate irregularities of the skin.

photophobia—fear of light.

photosensitivity—condition characterized by increased sensitivity to light and the effects of light, particularly sunlight, on the skin.

phymata (FYE-muh-tuh)—a small inflamed nodule on the skin.

phymatous (FYE-muh-tus)—pertaining to a phymata.

physical dependence—chemical dependence on an agent produced outside the body, which the body thinks it needs in order to function properly, despite that not being the case; the body then expresses physical conditions when the substance is withdrawn.

physiology—the study of body function.

phytotherapy—use of plants and herbs used for therapeutic purposes.

pilosebaceous (pye-loh-sye-**BAY**-shus) **unit**—the anatomical structure which comprises the hair follicle and accompanying sebaceous glands and arrector pili muscle. Together, this structure aids healing, skin moisture, product absorption, and sensation.

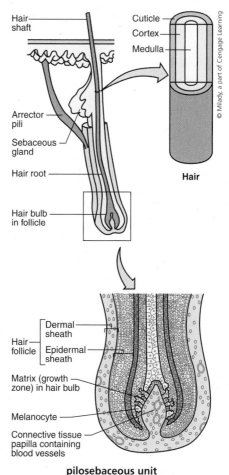

pilosebaceous unit

pineal gland—endocrine gland in the brain which secretes melatonin.

P–isoamyl Methoxycinnamate (eye-soh-AM-il meh-THOKS-ee-sin-num-ayt)—UV filter commonly found in sunscreens, or an additive in cosmetic preparations which offer UV protection.

pituitary (pih-TOO-ih-tayr-ee) **gland**—primary endocrine and growth-inducing gland found at the base of the brain and responsible for many functions, including growth.

plantar—referring to the area on the underside of the foot.

plaque—elevated solid lesion on the skin greater than 2 cm; formed by the coalescence of papules or nodules.

plaque psoriasis (PLAK soh-RYE-uh-sis)—type of psoriasis characterized by red, well-defined plaques on the cutaneous surfaces.

plasma—fluid portion of blood in which clotting elements and formed elements are suspended.

platelets—vital clotting cell of blood.

platysmal bands—bands of the neck which are a result of dynamic movement of the neck and jaw.

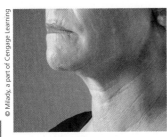

© Milady, a part of Cengage Learning

platysmal bands

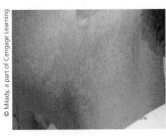

© Milady, a part of Cengage Learning

poikiloderma

pleural effusion—fluid leakage in the thoracic cavity.

plexus—a network of intersecting blood vessels, lymph vessels, or nerves; a web.

pneumonitis (noo-muh-NYE-tis)—a potentially dangerous inflammation of the lungs.

poikiloderma of Civatte (poy-kil-oh-DER-muhofsee-VAHT)—A common photoaging condition that is usually seen on sun-exposed necks and chests and consists primarily of vascular lesions and pigmentation.

poison—substance dangerous to life or well-being.

polyacrylamide—polymer used as a thickener in tanning products.

P

polychromatic—pertaining to many colors.

polymer—the result of synthetically combining small molecules into a new one.

polymorphic disease—a disease or condition that has multiple forms or subsets.

polypeptide—-a chain of amino acids.

polyphenols—a polymeric phenol compound.

polysaccharide—a group of carbohydrates.

popliteal (pop-LIT-ee-al) **veins**—deep veins located behind the knee.

porphyria (por-FEER-ee-uh)—a group of different disorders caused by abnormalities in production of heme, a substance that is important in the creation of blood and bone marrow. Heme contains iron and is a non-protein. Cutaneous porphyrias affect the skin with symptoms of blisters, itching, and swelling of the skin when exposed to sunlight.

porphyria cutanea tarda (por-FEER-ee-uh cue-TAYN-ee-uh TAR-duh)—genetic condition characterized by a disruption in normal polyphyrin metabolism.

porphyrins (POR-fuh-rins)—a compound that forms many important substances in the body including hemoglobin, a part of red blood cells that carries oxygen in the blood.

positive stool guaiac (GWYE-ak)—biologic test whose results indicate if blood is present in stool.

post-auricular—behind the ear.

post-herpetic neuralgia—nerve pain that occurs in a small percentage of patients that have suffered from herpes zoster (shingles). A pain remains in the healed area long after the blisters of the disease have cleared.

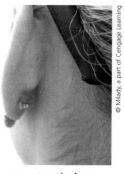

post-inflammatory hyperpigmentation (PIH)—A universal response of the skin, but it is more common in pigmented, darker skin. PIH can be caused by any inflammatory process, injury, surgery or laser/light therapy; the response of the melanocytes to injury.

© Milady, a part of Cengage Learning

post-auricular

post-mitotic cells—cells which have completed mitotic division.

post-operative——meaning after surgery.

post-thrombotic event—trauma caused to a vessel, resulting in inflammation.

Post-Traumatic Stress Disorder (PTSD)—anxiety condition which is the result of stress brought upon by a traumatic event.

potassium sulfate—synthetic product used to increase viscosity in cosmetics.

potent—strong and active; a substance with the ability to modify or change.

poultices—moist preparation placed on an aching or inflamed part of the body to relieve pain and inflammation.

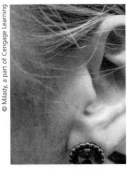

© Milady, a part of Cengage Learning

pre-auricular

pre-auricular—in front of the ear.

precipitate—a suspension that separates from a solution.

precocious puberty—early onset of puberty, including earlier than average presence of menstruation, pubic hair, and sexual desire. Early onset of puberty has psychosocial consequences for both males and females.

predisposed—possessing attributes which increase the likelihood of an event taking place.

prehypertension—state of being on the verge of having high blood pressure. Characterized by higher than recommended blood pressure and redness of the face.

prejudices—a negative or positive opinion based on ideas or facts that were known prior.

prescription—a doctor's order for a medication in order to remedy an illness or the symptoms of an illness. Regulated by the FDA, permission to dispense drugs is vital to the safety of the population at large. Prescriptions are encoded in medical shorthand and subsequently transcribed by pharmacists to ensure the safety of the public.

P

prescriptive devices—any medical devices that require specific education and regulatory requirements prior to use, and are governed by the FDA.

presentation—(1) the way a certain condition physically manifests itself (2) the way one appears; the physical manifestation of an idea or concept.

preservative—agent added to prevent microorganisms from forming on a food or drug.

pre-treatment—any process that will aid or facilitate a future procedure.

preventative maintenance (PM)—any strategy that is intended to reduce or eliminate the possibility of a disease, condition, or infection prior to its onset.

priapism (PRYE-ah-piz-em)—a prolonged abnormal erection without the presence of sexual desire.

primary colors—colors that are pure and not made from any other color combination. Rather, the colors from which all other colors on the visual spectrum are made: red, yellow, and blue.

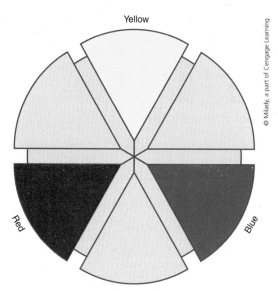

primary colors

© Milady, a part of Cengage Learning

primary hypercholesterolemia— the first in a series of events in which the affected individual presents with high cholesterol or a coronary artery disease diagnosis.

primary hypertension—the first in a series of events in which the affected individual presents with high blood pressure prior to intervention being taken.

primary infection—The first of a series of repeated presentations of a recurrent virus; usually has a different course that that of the subsequent infections. Commonly called the "initial outbreak or onset."

procerus (pro-SEER-us)—a muscle that connects the nose to the forehead.

progesterones (proh-JES-ter-ohns)—female sex hormone always involved in pregnancy and menstruation.

prognosis—the prediction of a disease's expected course from the diagnosis to the outcome.

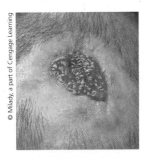

proliferative phase

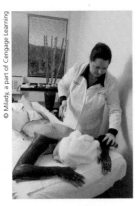

prone position

prolactin—hormone which stimulates the production of milk in women nursing infants.

proliferative phase—phase of wound-healing during which replacement of protective epithelial tissue occurs over the old wound site.

prone—when the body is lying with the face and chest turned downward.

prophylaxis (proh-fih-LAK-sis)—any treatment or technique whose intent is to prevent a disease or condition.

propionibacterium (proh-pee-on-eh-bak-TEER-ee-um)—bacterium thought to be responsible for acne and acne-related breakouts.

propolis (PROP-uh-lis)—originating from beeswax, a sun-protective agent also used for acne care due to its antibacterial qualities.

propylene glycol—a solvent, humectant, and moisturizing agent in esthetic preparations.

propyl parabens (PROH-pil PAR-eh-bens)—low-sensitivity, low-toxicity preservative.

prostaglandins (pros-tuh-GLAN-dins)—substances which resemble hormones but are called autocoids; act as intercellular or intracellular modulators. Play key roles in several bodily functions including blood pressure and muscle contraction.

prosthetic—replacement of a missing part with a man-made substitute.

protease (PROH-tee-ayz)—protein that can divide other proteins.

protein—class of complex compounds which are synthesized by all living creatures. Proteins are broken down into amino acids necessary for growth and development, and also for the rebuilding of tissue.

protein antibody—protein that is secreted into the blood or lymph in response to an antigenic stimulus, such as a bacterium, virus, parasite, or transplanted organ, and that neutralizes the antigen.

protein coagulation—peel frost; the phenomenon that occurs when certain peeling agents come in contact with proteins, like those found on the skin. In esthetics, used as timeline to indicate that the peel solution has achieved the optimal depth.

protein malnutrition—limited to poor intake or absorption of protein in one's diet.

proteinuria (proh-tee-in-YOO-ree-uh)—high levels of protein in the urine.

proteolysis—hydrolysis of protein; destruction of protein.

proton pump inhibitors—class of drugs which act as an anti-ulcer agent by restricting the acid production in the stomach. Used as a treatment for esophageal ulcers resulting from chronic acidosis.

protoplasm—thick fluid within cells that is the basis for all life. Contains the cytoplasm and nectoplasm.

protozoa—microorganisms; smallest organisms known.

pruritus (proo-RYE-tus)—itching.

pseudocollagen (soo-doh-KOL-uh-jen)—from plants; it acts as a moisturizing film on the skin in esthetic preparations.

pseudofolliculitis barbae (soo-doh-foh-lik-yoo-LYE-tis barb-ee)—a condition in which ingrown hairs produce an inflammatory reaction characterized by papules, pustules, and nodules; found after shaving.

pseudomonas (soo-doh-MOH-nas)—type of pathogen mostly found in the soil and in decomposing organic matter which is known to be resistant to antibiotics.

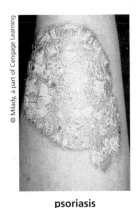

psoriasis

psoriasis (soh-RYE-uh-sis)—a chronic skin disease characterized by inflammation and white scaly patches.

psychological dependence—type of chemical dependency characterized by the affected individual thinking he or she needs a substance for normal functioning.

psychology—study of the mind and its relationship to behavioral patterns.

psychosis—most extreme cases of mental disturbance in which the affected individual has partially or totally lost touch with reality, either permanently or temporarily.

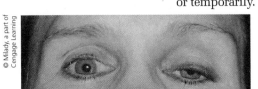

ptosis

ptosis (TOH-sis)—prolapse or sagging; drooping, especially of the upper eyelid from paralysis of the third cranial nerve. Consequence of improper administration of Botox.

pulmonary circulation—path deoxygenated blood takes to become oxygenated; in through the right ventricle, into the lungs through the pulmonary artery, and into the left atrium via the pulmonary vein.

pulmonary valve—valve that separates the pulmonary path from the right ventricle (*see* Fig. 2–17 on page 29).

pulse duration—the period of time in which a pulse of light is emitted during a laser treatment.

pulse width—*see* pulse duration.

pumping—the process whereby the energy source supplies energy to the active medium.

punctate keratitis (punk-tayt ker-ah-TYE-tis)—calluses resulting from prolonged and frequent exposure to friction.

purification—to take away impurities through thermal, chemical, or temporal means.

pustular psoriasis (PUS-tyool-ar soh-RYE-uh-sis)—type of psoriasis characterized by a pustular presentation.

P

pustule (PUS-tyool)—small, elevated, pus-filled abnormality of the skin common to many skin conditions, including but not limited to acne, eczema, impetigo, syphilis, smallpox, or poison ivy. They may or may not be accompanied by pruritis.

pustulosis (PUS-tyoo-low-sis)—any skin eruptions which are characterized by pustules.

pyruvic (pye-ROO-vik) **acid**—a phenol derivative; from sodium pyruvate. Has a very large molecule. Used for peeling and skin rejuvenation.

P

qi (CHEE)—*see* chi.

quadriceps—large muscle at the top of the thigh responsible for extending the leg.

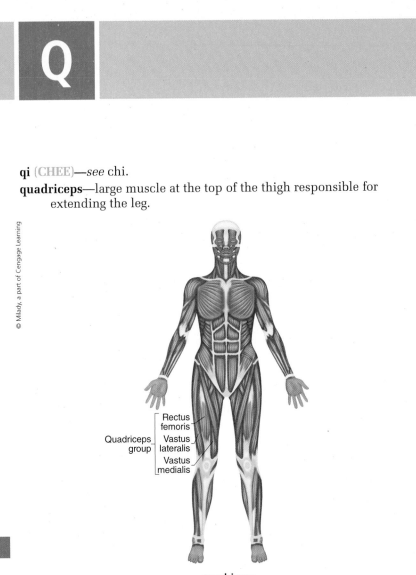

Quadriceps group ⎰ Rectus femoris
⎱ Vastus lateralis
⎰ Vastus medialis

quadriceps

quality assurance (QA)—a program that can cover all activities from design, development, production, installation, performance, and documentation in an effort to provide excellence to the consumer. QA is done so that a customer or client will be satisfied with the product or service and have a favorable opinion of the product or service. It identifies steps that may be taken along the way to ensure as much.

Radiance—commercial name for calcium hydroxyapatite (CAHA), a dermal filler. Typically used for augmentation of the cheeks and jawline. Can also be used as a volumizer on the sides of the face.

radio frequency (RF)—with regard to esthetics, used for promoting collagen growth. Frequently used in conjunction with skin rejuvenation devices such as RF-assisted lipoplasty. There are unipolar and bipolar devices available.

Raynaud's (ray-NOHZ) **disease**—condition characterized by abnormal vasoconstriction in the extremities, usually as a result of cold or stress; hands and fingers often blanch, turning pink or cyanotic. Common in women ages 18 to 30.

rebound hypoglycemia (hye-poh-glye-SEE-mee-uh)—phenomenon associated with decreased glucose levels following the external introduction of insulin into the body for individuals with diabetes. Symptoms include short-term lightheadedness, increased respiration, and fatigue.

rectus (REK-tus) **abdominis**—horizontally paired muscles running down the length of the abdomen.

recurrent infections—the second and subsequent infections of the active state of a virus; usually presents less intense than the primary infection.

reduction mammaplasty—type of breast surgery by which tissue is removed from the breast so that the breasts appear smaller. Commonly called a "breast reduction."

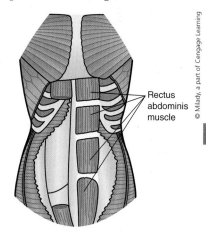

Rectus abdominis muscle

© Milady, a part of Cengage Learning

redundant skin—excess and unneeded flesh; the tissue usually removed during cosmetic surgeries.

re-epithelialization—the replacement of protective epithelial tissue.

reflexology—therapeutic method of relief in which certain pressure points are massaged in order to favorably influence other body functions.

reflux—backward pressure contrary to normal fluid flow.

regulations—rules decided by governing agencies or trade organizations as a uniform code of practice to ensure the well-being of their clientele.

remodeling phase—phase of wound healing during which collagen is assembled and discontinuous tissues are replaced.

renal failure—inability of the kidneys to function normally, with detrimental consequences to an individual's health and well-being.

Renova (REN-o-vah)—trade name for a preparation of tretinoin, which is meant specifically for anti-aging purposes. Recommended for patients with drier skin.

resorcinol (rih-ZOR-suh-nol)—equal parts hydroquinone and catechol; a peeling agent with similarities to phenol. Used for peeling and skin rejuvenation.

Restylane (RES-tuh-lin)—Trade name for hyaluronic acid dermal filler.

rete pegs (REE-tee)—anatomic feature which holds the dermis and epidermis together.

reticula—a netlike formation or structure of the skin; a network.

reticular dermis—sublayer of the dermis which connects the dermis to subcutaneous fat below it, and is home to the skin's appendages (nails, hair, glands) (*see* Fig. 2–40 on page 56).

reticulin—a water-soluble protein in the connective tissue framework of reticular tissue.

Retin-A—trade name for tretinoin, a topical keratolytic agent used to treat acne and reverse photodamage.

retinoic acid—oxidized form of vitamin A. Active ingredient in isotretinoin.

retinoids—class of drugs derived from vitamin A.

retinol—topical vitamin A derivative which must first convert to retinoic acid before it can be useful to the skin.

retinyl esters—topical products that are precursors to retinoic acid.

retinyl palmitate—topical vitamin A derivative which must first convert to retinoic acid before it can be useful to the skin. Also thought to be useful for collagen synthesis.

rheostat—a resistor designed to allow variation in resistance without breaking the electrical circuit.

rhinitis (rye-NYE-tis)—inflammation of the nasal mucosa.

rhinoplasty—surgical reshaping of the nose.

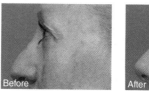
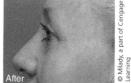

Before / After

rhinoplasty

rhytid (RYE-tide)—wrinkle of the skin associated with aging or dynamic movement.

rhytidectomy—cosmetic surgery intended to remove wrinkles or loose skin from the face; a facelift.

riboflavin (vitamin B)—used as an emollient in skin care products.

rigors—hardness or stiffness of the muscles.

ringworm—popular term for dermatomycosis due to

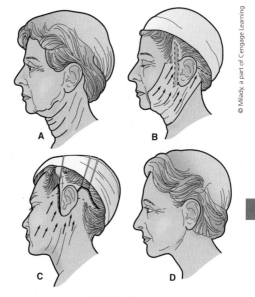

rhytidectomy

© Milady, a part of Cengage Learning

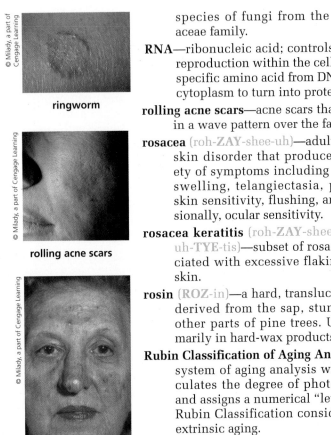

ringworm

rolling acne scars

rosacea

species of fungi from the Monili-
aceae family.

RNA—ribonucleic acid; controls protein
reproduction within the cell. Carries
specific amino acid from DNA to the
cytoplasm to turn into protein.

rolling acne scars—acne scars that appear
in a wave pattern over the face.

rosacea (roh-ZAY-shee-uh)—adult chronic
skin disorder that produces a variety of symptoms including redness,
swelling, telangiectasia, papules,
skin sensitivity, flushing, and, occasionally, ocular sensitivity.

rosacea keratitis (roh-ZAY-shee-uh ker-
uh-TYE-tis)—subset of rosacea associated with excessive flaking of the
skin.

rosin (ROZ-in)—a hard, translucent resin
derived from the sap, stumps, and
other parts of pine trees. Used primarily in hard-wax products.

Rubin Classification of Aging Analysis—a
system of aging analysis which calculates the degree of photodamage
and assigns a numerical "level." The
Rubin Classification considers only
extrinsic aging.

rugburn—slang for healing hot spots following a peeling treatment.

R

saccharide (SAK-uh-ride)—(1) groups of carbohydrates (2) a moisturizing agent.

safety bill of rights—original name for OSHA.

safety coordinator—specifically designated person in a business or organization who is responsible for enforcing regulatory codes of practice and updating OSHA Safety Manual as warranted.

Safety Manual—OSHA document which outlines the hazardous materials and equipment specific to each location, and the safety protocols for each.

sagittal (SADJ-ih-tal)—a vertical plane parallel to the central plane of the sagittal suture in the skull.

salicylate (sal-ih-SIL-ayt)—salt derivative of salicylic acid. Used as a chemical agent in sunscreens.

salicylate (sal-ih-SIL-ayt) **toxicity**—absorption of too much salicylic acid. Results in ear ringing, dehydration, and possible convulsions.

salicylic acid—beta-hydroxy acid derived from willow bark, used for chemical peels and topical skin care. It is oil-soluble and oil-dissolving, antimicrobial and anti-inflammatory, and a keratolytic. Acts by digesting the debris in follicles; good for the treatment of acne.

santalum alba (SAN-tal-um AL-ba)—sandalwood essential oil; for dry, dehydrated skin.

SAPHO syndrome—a chronic disorder that involves the skin, bone, and joints. SAPHO is an acroynm for synovitis, acne, pustulosis, hyperostosis, and osteitis. All of these diseases can and do occur together in this very severe form of acne.

saturation index—*see* Langlier index.

scale—skin condition characterized by epidermal thickening.

scar—mark left in the skin, or on an internal organ, as a result of deep tissue trauma. Scars are a result of injury, disease, or medical procedures. They are permanent and are often considered unsightly by those who have them.

schizophrenia (skit-suh-FREE-nee-uh)—personality disorder characterized by a disassociation from social experience and limited social range.

sclerodactyly (sklehr-oh-DAK-teh-lee)—pertaining to hardening of the skin on the fingers and toes.

scleroderma (sklehr-oh-DER-ma)—chronic tissue condition characterized by the hardening of the skin as well as internal organs, including the heart, kidneys, lungs, and gastrointestinal tract.

sclerose—to harden; commonly used when describing the arteries, for example, atherosclerosis.

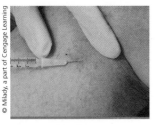

© Milady, a part of Cengage Learning

sclerotherapy

sclerotherapy—injection into a vein of a chemical irritant that causes irritation and fibrosis of the vein. Later, the vein will absorb the irritant and will not be visible. Used to treat varicose veins, hemorrhoids, or esophageal varices.

scotch hose—a hose similar to a fire hose used in hydrotherapy. Utilizes higher-pressure water emissions to cleanse and massage.

SCULPTRA—product used to remedy facial lipodystrophy in patients with HIV; used off-label to treat aging lipodystrophy.

SD alcohol—denatured alcohol for cosmetic use.

seabather's eruption—Papules and pruritis which appear on the skin shortly after swimming in ocean waters. The lesions will crust over and resolve spontaneously within a week or two. Likely caused by a waterborne pathogen common in North American waterways.

sea scrub—esthetic treatment that utilizes sea-based minerals to increase circulation, exfoliate, and moisturize to reveal a healthier skin tone.

seaweed extract—originating from one of the many varieties of seaweed; strong healing properties.

seaweed wraps—skin treatment that includes application of a seaweed mask followed by a thermal blanket to seal in heat.

sebaceous (seh-BAY-shus)—pertaining to oil or sebum on the skin.

sebaceous (seh-BAY-shus) **glands**—a small gland usually located next to the hair follicle in the dermis that releases

S

fatty liquids onto the hair follicle to soften hair and skin.

sebaceous (seh-BAY-shus) **hyperplasia**—a common condition of enlarged sebaceous glands of the face.

seborrhea (seb-oh-REE-ah)—condition characterized by excessive sebaceous secretion.

seborrheic dermatitis (seb-oh-REE-ik der-mah-TYE-tis)—chronic inflammatory disease of the skin which presents with red itchy patches, particularly in areas with a high concentration of sebum glands. Unknown etiology.

seborrheic keratosis (seb-oh-REE-ik kerr-ah-TOH-tis)—superficial, benign lesion consisting of proliferating epidermal cells enclosing horn cysts, usually appearing on the face, trunk, or extremities in adulthood.

sebum (SEE-bum)—the semifluid viscous secretion of the sebaceous glands, consisting chiefly of fat, keratin, and cellular material. Commonly referred to as "oil." It is sebum which combines with other debris and results in acne breakouts in the presence of P.acnes bacterium.

secondary colors—made by blending two of the primary colors (*see* illustration on next page).

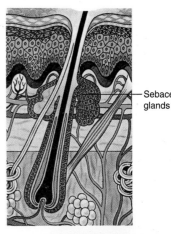

Sebaceous glands

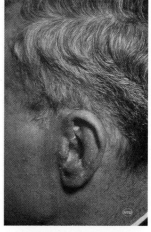

seborrhea dermatitis

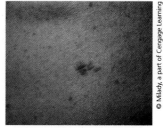

seborrhea keratosis

S

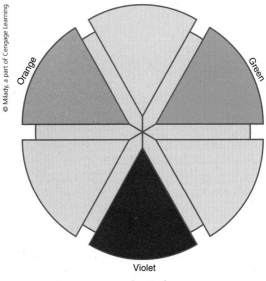

secondary colors

secretion—the process of producing and discharging substances from glands.

selective photothermolysis (foh-toh-thurm-uh-LYE-sis)—the specific targeting of one color on the spectrum for heat destruction while leaving surround colors untouched. The main process by which laser hair removal is performed.

select serotonin reuptake inhibitors (SSRIs)—type of antidepressant which allows for more available use of the neurotransmitter serotonin.

selenium (sih-LEE-nee-um)—a mineral resembling sulfur. Helps protect the skin from solar-induced skin cancers. Taken orally in supplements or applied topically as an additive in cosmetic solutions.

semilunar (sem-ee-LOO-nar) **valves**—valves of the aortic and pulmonary arteries that prevent backflow from arteries into the ventricles.

seminiferous (sem-ee-NIF-er-us)—producing semen; tubules of the testes.

senescence (sih-NES-ens)—growing old; aging.

septisol—antibacterial cleansing agent for the skin.

septum—creating two areas; a wall; the part of the nose that divides the two nostrils.

seropurulent (ser-oh-PYOO-reh-lent)—a combination of serum and pus.

serosanguinous (ser-oh-san-GWIN-ee-us) **fluid**—fluid containing both blood and serum.

serotonin—neurotransmitter whose abnormal production or absorption is associated with many mental illnesses, including depression, anxiety disorders, and personality disorders.

serpiginous (ser-PIJ-in-us)—creeping from one location to another location; for example, mast cancers are considered serpiginous because they can spread easily from one organ to another.

serum—blood plasma that is yellow in color.

shading—blending or fading of color or hair from a more- to less-saturated area.

sharps container—a closed container used to dispose of contaminated needles so they can be isolated for proper disposal.

shinbone—the flat surface of the bone immediately under the skin on the front of the lower leg extending from the knee to the ankle.

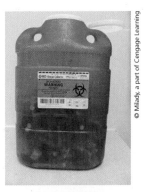

sharps container

shingles—condition characterized by acute herpetic eruptions on the skin caused by a recurrent infection of the herpes zoster virus. Typically found on the trunk but can occur on the face and in the eye.

side effect—an action or effect of a drug or a treatment which is expected in some but is not the general rule. Not to be confused with more severe consequences. Often considered by the patient as being more endurable than the originally treated condition, for example, nausea or short-term pain.

silicone—semi-organic polymers characterized as having extreme water

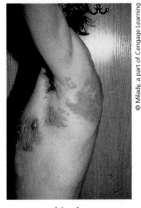

shingles

repellency, thermal stability, and lubricity. Used in a variety of esthetic treatments to increase volume, for example, lip augmentation or breast augmentation.

sinus—a pouch or cavity in any organ or tissue. Most commonly associated with the nasal cavity.

sitz bath—a therapeutic hydrotherapy treatment which increases blood flow to abdominal regions. Commonly used by mothers after giving vaginal birth or for hemorrhoid relief.

Attached to bones or, for some facial muscles, to skin

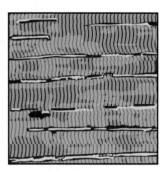

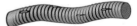

Single, very long, cylindrical, multinucleate cells with very obvious striations

skeletal muscles

skeletal muscles—type of voluntary muscles which surround, protect, and move the skeletal system.

skin condition—fundamental skin classification in which an individual's skin is grouped according to the degree of moisture retention and/or its reaction to products or environment. Skin condition is classified as being normal, dry, oily, or a combination.

skin graft—medical procedure used to repair or replace injured skin. Live, healthy skin is removed from one area and used to replace injured tissue elsewhere.

skin turgor—the flexibility of the skin; especially descriptive after a chemical peel. For example, the skin turgor is harder after a TCA peel.

skin typing—a more detailed skin classification which gives indications as to how a certain skin type will react to various treatment conditions. There are many different means of skin typing, and each has its own merits. The treatment being performed and the individual will determine which method is most appropriate.

skin wellness—active processes taken by an individual to ensure skin health over time. Skin wellness includes choosing to eat nutritious foods, actively protecting skin from harmful effects of the sun, and adherence to a prescribed regimen designed to a specific individual.

sloughing (SLUF-ing)—the casting off of skin, feathers, hair, or horns.

small saphenous (suh-FEE-nus) **veins**—smaller of the superficial and deep veins, clearly noticeable on the legs. Occasionally the object of sclerotherapy or surgical vein therapy.

smooth muscles—type of nonstriated muscles which line and function to aid the involuntary operation of hollow cavity organs, such as the stomach and bladder.

social isolation—complete retreat from others.

sociology—the study of humans and the collective groupings they form to enhance or perpetuate their future existence.

social phobias—a fear of public places or interacting with other people, that is so intense that it results in the need to avoid that thing in a manner which interferes with normal functioning.

social withdrawal—pulling away from friends and peers.

sodium benzoate—antiseptic and preservative for cosmetic preparations.

sodium bicarbonate—an alkaline substance; used to adjust skin pH in peeling or in skin care products. Commonly known as baking soda.

sodium chloride—in esthetics, used as an astringent or a thickener; common table salt.

sodium hydroxide—agent for soap-making; also called caustic soda or lye.

sodium lauryl sulfate—common ingredient in household detergents and soaps. Used as an emulsifier.

sodium silicate—a component found in the clays kaolin and bentonite. Active ingredient in many facials and masks.

soft tissue edema (eh-DEE-muh)—a collection of fluids in the soft tissues, including the skin, muscles, and organs.

solar lentigines (lehn-TIHJ-eh-neez)—spots on the skin, specifically caused by repeated sun exposure. One of the more common skin complaints of esthetic clients, this condition

S

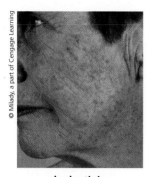

solar lentigines

can be treated with bleaching agents, laser treatments, and other noninvasive treatments.

soleus (SOH-lee-us)—long muscle situated under the "calf" muscles.

sorbic acid—commonly found in berries, a humectant and preservative in esthetic and cosmetic preparations.

sorbitol—a humectant and binding agent in esthetic and cosmetic preparations.

spasticity—pertaining to spasms or uncontrollable muscle movement.

specific phobias—fear of a specific thing which results in the need to avoid that specific thing to such a degree that it interferes with normal functioning.

specular reflection—opposite reflection, as when looking in a mirror.

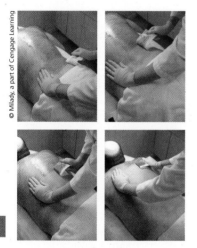

speed waxing

speed waxing—technique in which wax is applied and rapidly removed with muslin strips. This technique is best used with fearful clients and often involves coaching the client.

SPF—*see* sun protection factor.

sphincter (SFINK-ter)—circular muscle, controls an opening.

spider veins—*see* telangiectasia.

splattering—the appearance of tiny black spots, which are singed hairs, in hair follicles; caused by laser treatments. Not a permanent phenomenon.

splenomegaly (splee-noh-MEG-uh-lee)—condition characterized by the enlargement of the spleen.

S

spontaneous emission—the process whereby an excited atom, after holding extra energy for a fraction of a second, releases its energy as another photon, then falls back to its grounded state.

spot size—the width of a laser beam on its intended target.

squalene (SKWAY-leen)—from shark liver oil; lubricant, compatible with human skin, used in esthetic and cosmetic preparations. Should not be used on vegetarians or vegans.

squamous (SKWAY-mus) **cell carcinoma (SCC)**—malignant tumor of the epithelial cells. Frequently occurs on the ears, nose, and lips. Can be a result of prolonged sun exposure and a conversion of actinic keratosis.

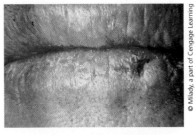

© Milady, a part of Cengage Learning

squamous cell carcinoma

staphylococcus (staf-ih-loh-KOK-sus)—common genus of bacterium responsible for many skin implications. By many accounts, the healthy, uncompromised human skin has hundreds of millions of these infectious bacteria on it at any given moment. If it enters the body, these bacteria can be responsible for a variety of conditions with both limited and detrimental consequence. Most significant is MRSA. Clients with MRSA require immediate medical attention.

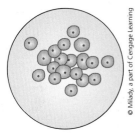

© Milady, a part of Cengage Learning

staphylococcus

static—occurring without the aid of movement; occurring independently.

static rhytids (RYE-tides)—wrinkling that occurs without reference to facial movement.

steareth (stee-AR-eth) **compounds**—solubilizers and co-emulsifiers.

stearic (stee-AR-ik) **acid**—emulsifier and thickener from vegetable fats.

stem cells—unspecialized cell which gives rise to a specific specialized cell.

S

sterilize—the destruction of all microbial life by heat, chemical, or gas to render them unable to reproduce.

sternocleidomastoids (ster-noh-klye-noh-MAS-toyds)—pair of muscles in the neck which serve to flex and rotate the head.

steroid—any number of fat-soluble organic compounds with specific clinical uses. Produced synthetically for medicinal and non-medicinal purposes. Often used for off-label and illegal purposes as a performance-enhancing agent in athletes or bodybuilders.

steroid-dependent dermatoses—condition of the skin in which the long-term overuse of topical steroid creams causes the skin to require continued usage to keep the offending condition away.

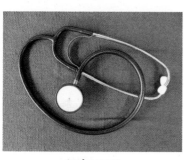

© Milady, a part of Cengage Learning

stethoscope

stethoscope—device used to magnify the sound of a beating heart, respirations of the lungs, or bowel sounds.

Stevens-Johnson syndrome—a life-threatening, major hypersensitivity reaction. Not the same as erythema multiforme minor.

stippling—dotting or dabbing of color in application using short strokes, as in permanent or applied makeup.

stomion (STOH-mee-on)—the median point of the oral slit when the lips are closed.

strabismus (strah-BIZ-mus)—eye disorder in which the optic axes in either eye cannot focus on the same object.

stratified epithelium—layers of tissue that lack blood vessels; acts as a surface barrier. Very superficial injuries which do not bleed only penetrate this layer of the skin.

stratum basale (STRAH-tum bay-SAY-lee)—the lowest sublayer of the epidermis. The stratum basale (basal layer) houses germinal cells, pigmentary cells, and regenerating cells for all layers of the epidermis.

stratum corneum (STRAH-tum KOR-nee-um)—the top sublayer of the epidermis; that layer that is exposed to the environment.

S

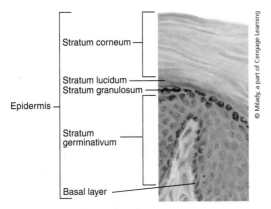

stratum layers

stratum granulosum (STRAH-tum gran-yoo-LOH-sum)—the granular sublayer of the epidermis found at the bottom of the horny zone.

stratum lucidum (STRAH-tum LOO-sih-dum)—sublayer of the epidermis characterized by the appearance of granules and the disappearance of the nucleus within the skin cells.

stratum spinosum (STRAH-tum spye-NO-sum)—the superior layer of the stratum germinativum; named for its shape and spiny, thorn-like protrusions; also known as the "prickle cell layer".

streptococcus (strep-toh-KOK-suhs)—genus of pathogenic bacterium which occurs in pairs or chains, many species of which destroy red blood cells and cause various diseases in humans.

striated—lined or ribbed.

strip method—technique for hair removal that uses a fabric strip rather than sugar or wax.

styptic (STIP-tik)—astringent for bleeding; styptic pencil.

sub—meaning below; as in subcutaneous.

subacute—not acute but not chronic; limited recurrence.

subcutaneous—beneath the skin.

subcutaneous fat—layer found just below the dermis (*see* illustration on next page).

subcutaneous mycoses—fungal infections which are localized to the exterior layers of the dermis in the skin and its appendages.

S

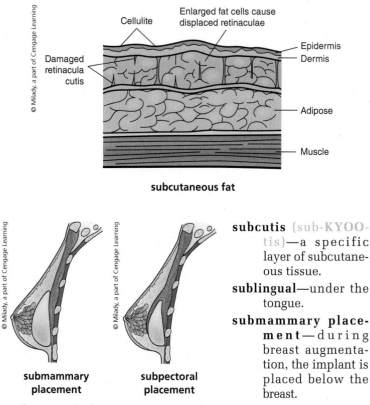

subcutaneous fat

subcutis (sub-KYOO-tis)—a specific layer of subcutaneous tissue.

sublingual—under the tongue.

submammary placement—during breast augmentation, the implant is placed below the breast.

subpectoral placement—during breast augmentation, the implant is placed below the pectoral muscle.

sudoriferous (soo-doh-RIF-er-us) **glands**—the skin's sweat glands. Situated in the skin just under the subcutaneous tissue. These sweat glands help to control the body's temperature.

sugaring—a type of hair removal process (*see* illustration on next page).

sugar wax—a product for hair removal; mostly made of sugar.

sun protection factor (SPF)—measurement of time an individual can be in the sun with protection from a sunscreen and not burn. SPF varies from one individual to the next depending on skin type.

sunscreen—any agent which protects the skin from harmful UVA and UVB light. In turn, it helps protect skin from photodamage, including skin cancers, dyschromia, and other photodamage such as aging. Sunscreens block or absorb harmful rays either by physical or chemical means.

supercilious (soo-per-SIL-ee-us)—expressing superiority or disdain.

superficial musculoaponeurotic (mus-kyoo-loh-ap-eh-noo-ROT-ik)—**system**—composed of muscle and fibrous tissue.

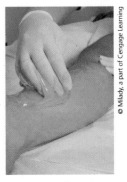

sugaring

superficial mycoses—usually result from the introduction of vegetative matter to an open wound; infection is limited to the dermis.

superficial peel—peel depth which extends into the stratum granulosum. These peels are not intended to cause bleeding or scarring and have limited down-time.

super-wet liposuction—type of liposuction during which large amounts of fluids containing lidocaine and other medications and fluids are injected into fatty tissues prior to suction.

supination—to rotate a joint a complete 180 degrees. For example, rotating the wrist so that the palm faces up and then faces down.

supine position—lying with the front or face upward.

suppurate—to form or discharge pus.

supra—above.

supraorbital—above the eye socket.

supraspinatus (soo-prah-spye-NAY-tus)—rotator cuff muscle.

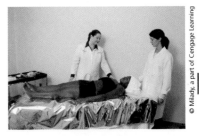

supine position

surfactant—surface-active agent that lowers surface tension. Commonly found in esthetic and cosmetic preparations, particularly cleansers.

symphisis (SIM-fuh-sis) **of the mandible**—the areas where the jawbone is fused together.

synapse—the junction across which a nerve impulse passes from the terminal to the neuron or neuromuscular junction.

syncope (SIN-koh-pee)—a momentary loss of blood flow to the brain resulting in unconsciousness; fainting.

syringoma (ser-in-GOH-muh)—a tumor of the sweat glands.

systemic antifungals—systemic medications intended to resolve fungal conditions. They are ingested orally and distributed via the bloodstream.

systemic circulation—blood and lymph circulation from the heart, through the arteries, to tissue and cells, and back to the heart by way of the veins.

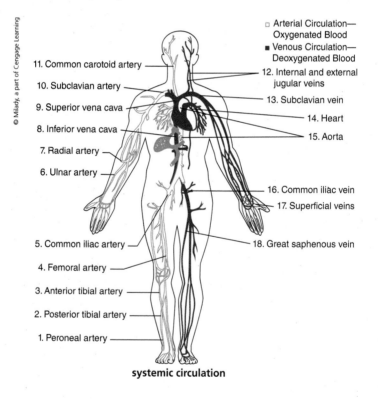

© Milady, a part of Cengage Learning

□ Arterial Circulation—
   Oxygenated Blood
■ Venous Circulation—
   Deoxygenated Blood

11. Common carotoid artery
10. Subclavian artery
9. Superior vena cava
8. Inferior vena cava
7. Radial artery
6. Ulnar artery
5. Common iliac artery
4. Femoral artery
3. Anterior tibial artery
2. Posterior tibial artery
1. Peroneal artery

12. Internal and external jugular veins
13. Subclavian vein
14. Heart
15. Aorta
16. Common iliac vein
17. Superficial veins
18. Great saphenous vein

systemic circulation

S

systemic lupus—chronic autoimmune disease of connective tissue which results in injury to various affected tissue. Identified by the telltale "butterfly" mask over the nose.

systemic mycoses—a fungus which affects the internal organs.

systemic toxicity—a poison causing widespread damage.

systolic (sis-TOL-ik)—period in the cycle of the heartbeat in which the heart is contracting.

S

tachycardia (tak-ee-KAR-dee-uh)—abnormally rapid heartbeat; usually over 100 beats per minute. The average is 80 beats per minute.

tallow—occlusive agent; primary agent in soaps, cultivated from fatty animal tissue; fatty tissue often used in candle manufacturing.

tannic acid—a brownish yellow coloration agent found in plants and used as an astringent in esthetic and cosmetic preparations.

tannins—astringent derived from tannic acid.

tartaric (tar-TAYR-ik) **acid**—alpha-hydroxy acid derived from grapes and used in esthetic and cosmetic preparations.

tatau—basis of the word "tattoo." Originates from the Polynesian word for "to mark something.".

TCA—*see* trichloracetic acid.

technique-sensitive—in esthetics, refers to the inability of one person to exactly replicate the results of another even when exact protocols and processes are observed. Individual variations in pressure or style will produce varying results.

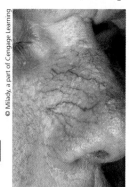

© Milady, a part of Cengage Learning

telangiectasia

telangiectasia (tel-an-jee-ek-TAY-zee-uh)—dilation of something previously small, as in a blood vessel. Also known as spider veins.

telangiectasia (tel-an-jee-ek-TAY-zee-uh) **matting**—an irritation of the blood vessels typically resulting from a sclerosing agent which causes the vessels to appear as a pink swatch over the treated area.

telogen phase—stage of hair growth during which the hair is at rest.

temperature—unit of measurement of heat. Expressed in degrees Celsius (C) or Fahrenheit (F).

temporalis—muscle that lowers the jaw.

tendons—fibrous and tough fiber that connects muscle tissue to a bone or joint.

terminal—any illness that will result in death; an end; the point where something ends or starts a new process.

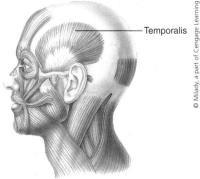
Temporalis

© Milady, a part of Cengage Learning

terminal hair—hair found on the scalp, arms, legs, axillae, and pubic area.

terminal sterilization—amidst the transition from nonsterile to sterile.

terpinol—active ingredient of tea tree oil.

tertiary colors—made by mixing two secondary colors or by mixing a primary with the secondary color next to it. Pertains to the color wheel and applied or permanent makeup.

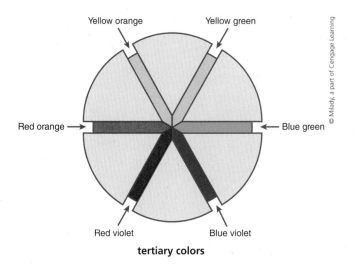

tertiary colors

tetrasodium—preservative and chelating agent used in esthetic and cosmetic preparations.

TEWL—*see* transepidermal water loss.

T

thalassemia (thal-ah-SEE-mee-ah)—genetic condition characterized by defective red blood cell production, resulting in oxygen deficiency.

thalassotherapy (thal-uh-soh-THAYR-uh-pee)—the therapeutic use of the beneficial effects of seawater.

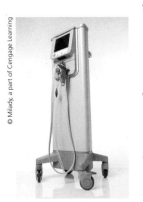

Thermage

therapeutic program—skin treatment program which is assisted by prescriptions, vitamins, and sunscreens in order to achieve a positive and healthy outcome for the skin's overall health and appearance.

Thermage—non-invasive radio frequency technology used to improve facial appearance through the improvement of collagen growth.

thermal relaxation time—the time it takes skin tissue to cool following heating associated with thermal laser therapies.

thermolysis—the use of heat to remove or destroy tissue or offending agents.

thiamine (THYE-uh-min)—*see* vitamin B complex.

thickener—ingredients in esthetic and cosmetic preparations used to improve the solidity or viscosity of a product.

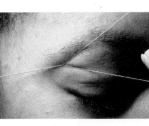

threading

threading—the use of thin strips of material to remove hair by rolling them across a particular area with the intent that the rotary motion will attach to the hairs and pluck them from the root.

thrombocytopenia (throm-boh-sye-TOH-sis)—abnormal decrease in blood platelet levels.

thrombosis (throm-BOH-sis)—formation or presence of one or more blood clots that may partially or completely block a vessel.

thymosin (THYE-moh-sin)—hormones responsible for the production of T-cells, white blood cells which are vital to the immune system.

thymus (THYE-mus)—organ responsible for the production of T-cells.

T

thyroid—an endocrine gland located in the neck; secretes a variety of active substances vital to normal bodily function. Over- or underproduction of these secretions result in many caustic problems for affected individuals which are difficult to pinpoint. (*See* Figs. 2–13 to 2–15 on pages 23–25.)

thyrotropic hormone—hormone which stimulates the thyroid gland.

thyroxine (thye-ROK-seen)—main thyroid hormone responsible for metabolism and growth.

tibial vein—deep vein which runs along side of the tibia. Vital for lower extremity blood supply.

tibialis anterior—long muscle which runs the length of the tibia and maneuvers the foot.

tic—a spastic muscle contraction, usually involving the face or hands.

tincture—herb prepared with alcohol and water, used in esthetic and cosmetic and medicinal preparations.

tinea capitis (TIN-ee-ah KAP-ih-tis)—fungal infection of the scalp.

tinea corporis (TIN-ee-ah KOR-puh-ris)—fungal infection affecting the body, commonly called "ringworm."

tinea cruris (TIN-ee-ah KROOR-is)—fungal infection of the area surrounding the genitalia (also called "jock itch").

tinea faciei (TIN-ee-ah FEY-shee-eye)—fungal infection affecting the face.

tinea (TIN-ee-ah) **manuum**—fungal infection affecting the hands.

tinea pedis (TIN-ee-ah PED-ee-ah)—fungal infection affecting the feet. Also called "athlete's foot."

tinea versicolor (TIN-ee-ah VUR-sih-kul-er)—fungal skin infection affecting the trunk which presents as macular patches appearing lighter than surrounding tissue.

tinnitus (tih-NYE-tus)—ringing in the ears.

titanium dioxide—non-chemical physical sunscreen which scatters light rather than absorbing or filtering it.

tocopherol (toh-KOF-er-ol)—vitamin E.

toner—a cosmetic product intended for individuals with combination or normal skin with the intention of controlling sebum and improving the condition the skin. Typically used in the T-zone for individuals with combination skin.

Can also be used as a clarifier for all clients to ensure all the makeup is removed at the end of the day.

topical—a medication, lotion, ointment, or moisturizer applied to the skin.

topical antifungals—any antifungal medication which is applied topically on the skin.

topical isotretinoin (eye-soh-trih-TIN-oyn)—*see* isotretinoin.

tortuous (TOR-choo-us)—taking a twisting, nonlinear path.

total body surface area (TBSA)—used when calculating the percentage of the body burned in an accident or otherwise. Not related to sunburns.

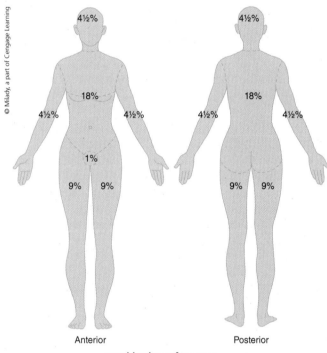

© Milady, a part of Cengage Learning

total body surface area

toxic epidermal necrolysis—*see* epidermal necrosis.

toxicology—the study of poisons and their effects on the human body.

toxin—a poisonous agent which has the potential to cause damage to an individual or their functional processes.

tragus (TRAY-gus)—cartilage in front of the ear; the point of cartilage (*see* illustration on next page).

transduction—means by which bacteria or viruses undergo genetic recombination, carrying DNA from one bacterium to another.

transepidermal water loss (TEWL)—the process by which the body constantly loses water via evaporation.

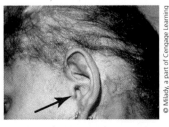

tragus

transverse—crosswise to something else.

trapezius—two flat fleshy muscles which span either side of the upper back, allowing for movement of the head and shoulders.

traverse abdominals—innermost layer of abdominal muscles.

treatment—administration of remedies or therapies with the intent of curing a condition or managing its symptoms.

treatment consequence—*see* consequence.

treatment history—a period of time long enough to assess results and whether the prescribed treatment modality is having the desired effect or if another course is necessary.

treatment plan—plan of action for patient care. Involves the pre-treatment case plan, the actual esthetic treatment, and the follow-up home care plan.

treatment table—the platform specifically designed to perform esthetic treatments.

trend—a momentary tendency toward one proclivity versus another based on the direction of others.

tricep brachii (BRAY-kee-eye)—large muscle that runs along the underside of the upper arm, acting to extend the arm.

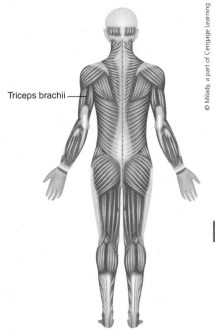

Triceps brachii

T

triclosan (try-KLOH-san)—preservative and antibacterial used in cosmetic preparations.

tricuspid valve—heart valve which prevents backflow between the right atrium and right ventricle (*see* Fig. 2–17 on page 29).

tricyclics—class of psychotropic drugs; among the most commonly prescribed for certain mild cases of depression or anxiety.

triethanolamine (TRY-eth-uh-nol-uh-meen) **(TEA)**—emulsifier in cosmetic preparations.

trigeminal neuralgia (try-JEM-ih-nul new-RAL-jee-uh)—nerve pain along the nerves of the face.

trigger—an event or set of circumstances which causes an otherwise dormant virus or condition to reactivate.

triticum vulgare (TRY-tih-kum vul-GAY-ree)—wheat germ oil.

tubules—a very small tube.

tumesce, tumesced—to inject fluid into; swollen with fluid.

tumescent anesthesia—delivery technique through an injection or with the assistance of a pump. A diluted Lidocaine and epinephrine solution typically used during liposuction, it is injected for pain control and reduction of bleeding.

tumescent liposuction—a technique where Xylocaine and other medications are injected into the surgical site before the liposuction is performed.

tummy tuck—*see* abdominoplasty.

tumor—abnormal growth of cells. Can be either benign or malignant.

turbinates—bones in the nose, shaped like a cone.

turgor (TER-ger)—skin's flexibility. Lack of flexibility presents as loose skin and wrinkling.

type 1 diabetes—type of diabetes in which the body cannot produce insulin, or insulin is ineffective, resulting in the need for external supplies of insulin to be introduced. Also called childhood diabetes.

type 2 diabetes—type of diabetes in which the body cannot properly utilize insulin, resulting in the need for monitoring or diet and exercise in addition to medication.

tyrosine (TYE-roh-seen)—amino acid; while controversial, topical applications will stimulate melanin synthesis.

ubiquinone (yoo-BIK-wih-nohn)—*see* coenzyme Q10.

ulcer—loss of epidermis and dermis in internal tissues.

ultrasound—the use of sound waves to create an image of soft tissue. This technique is used to diagnose soft tissue irregularities.

ultraviolet—electromagnetic radiation with wavelengths shorter than the visible spectrum of light. UVA and UVB wavelengths range from 180 to 400 nm.

umbilicate—(1) possessing a central depression (2) having an umbilical cord.

umbilicus—the belly button.

unguent (UNG-gwunt)—a salve or ointment used to promote healing.

unicellular—pertaining to only one cell.

United States Pharmacopoeia (USP)—protocol for pharmacists practicing in the United States, specifically a compendium of drug standards, including assays and tests for determining drug strength and purity.

universal precautions—preventative actions taken to prevent the transmission of pathogens; involves the use of protective procedures and equipment, such as gloves and masks.

unrealistic expectation—a belief that a certain outcome is possible, regardless of merit or circumstance.

upper facelifts—cosmetic procedure involving areas above the jawline and below the forehead.

urea (yoo-REE-uh)—primary acid contained in urine. It is primarily a protein metabolizer.

urticaria (ur-tih-KAYR-ree-uh)—*see* urticaria pigmentosa.

USP—*see* United States Pharmacopoeia.

urticaria pigmentosa (ur-tih-KAYR-ree-uh pig-men-TOH-suh)— allergic reactions such as hives with a large number of mast cells.

valproates (val-PROH-ayts)—anticonvulsive drugs which are meant to limit the frequency and severity of spastic activity.

Valtrex—antiviral most commonly used to suppress HSV-1 and HSV-2.

varices (VAYR-ih-seez)—abnormally dilated or bulging veins.

varicella (var-ih-SEL-uh)—virus which is responsible for both chickenpox and herpes zoster.

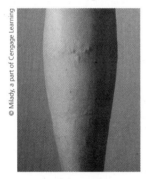

© Milady, a part of Cengage Learning

varicose veins

varicose veins—condition characterized by swollen veins, most commonly in the legs.

vascular—pertaining to veins.

vasodilation—an increase in the flow capacity of veins as a result of the widening of the blood vessels.

vasopressin—antidiuretic hormone which increases blood pressure.

vegetable oil—oil from a plant.

vellus—fine, short hair with no pigment, found mainly on women's faces; also referred to as "peach fuzz."

venous lakes—skin condition characterized by dilated veins which occur on sun-damaged skin.

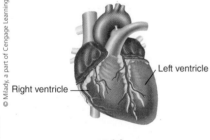

© Milady, a part of Cengage Learning

Right ventricle
Left ventricle

ventricles

ventricles—the lower chambers of the heart that force blood either to the lungs for oxygenation, or out to the body.

ventricular arrhythmia (VEN-trik-yoo-ler ah-RITH-mee-uh)—

irregular heartbeat which has its origin in the ventricular chambers of the heart.

ventricular tachycardia (VEN-trik-yoo-ler tak-ee-KAR-dee-uh)—abnormally rapid heartbeat that is caused by the pumping of the ventricular chambers of the heart.

venulectasis (VEN-u-la-ta-sha)—*see* telangiestasia.

venules (VEN-yools)—small blood vessels with thin walls that receive blood from capillaries and convey it into veins.

vermillion border—The pinkish-colored boundary of the upper and lower lip representing the border oral mucosa; forms the cupid's bow on upper lip.

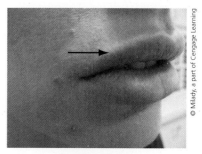

vermillion border

vertigo—sensation of moving through space or of having objects rotate around oneself independently. Often (erroneously) synonymous with dizziness.

very superficial peels—peel depths which do not achieve erythema or flaking. Used to achieve a fresh look to the skin.

vesicles—fluid-filled containers on the skin's surface.

vesiculation—the process of forming blisters.

vichy (VISH-ee) **shower**—an overhead stream of adjustable pressured water used in esthetic body treatments.

virilism—the presence of male-patterned hair growth and other male secondary sex characteristics in women.

virology—the study of viruses and their progression.

virus—a pathogenic unicellular particle, much smaller than bacteria, which occupies the DNA of a host cell, replicates, and spreads to other similar organisms.

viscosity—pourability or stickiness.

vitamin A—necessary for the regeneration of skin cells; vitamin A esters convert to retinoic acid in the skin. Vitamin A improves the skin's tone, texture, and density.

vitamin B—complex of vitamins found mostly in grains necessary to a variety of bodily functions. Applied to cosmetic preparations, although currently controversial as to how or if vitamin B can penetrate the skin surface.

V

vitamin C—antioxidant which is a necessary factor for the formation of collagen in connective tissue and maintenance of integrity of intercellular cement.

vitamin D—vital to the epidermal process; seems to improve the tone and texture of the skin.

vitamin E—antioxidant which has been shown to deactivate free radicals. However, the exact mechanism whereby it functions is unknown.

vitamin E linoleate (leh-NOH-lee-ayt)—synthetic vitamin E.

vitamin F—linoleic acid; for dry skin.

vitamin H—biotin; for acne treatment.

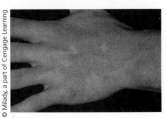

vitiligo

vitamin P—possible protection from collagen destruction.

vitiligo (vit-ih-LYE-goh)—disease of the melanocytes, resulting in patches of hypopigmentation.

vitreous hemorrhage—bleeding in the eye.

voluntarily—acting upon free will, without instinct or coercion.

V

waterborne infections—the passage of microbial agents and pathogens in heated water. Common in spas, gyms, and public pools.

watt—the unit of power produced by a current of 1 ampere acting across a potential difference of 1 volt.

wavelength—the distance between two consecutive peaks or troughs in a wave.

wax—generic term for any water-repellent esters.

wheal—accumulation of localized edema, typical of urticaria.

white blood cell—*see* leukocyte.

white lip—the external lip which encases the muscles below and acts to move the encased muscle.

W/O—water in oil (emulsion).

wood's lamp—a black light that reveals variation in skin color according to skin condition and is used during the skin analysis portion of a facial treatment.

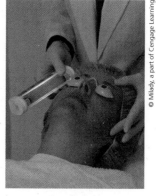

© Milady, a part of Cengage Learning

wound—a disruption of normal tissue which results from pathological processes beginning internally or externally to the involved organ. *See* insult.

wound healing—the restoration of tissue continuity following injury or trauma.

wood's lamp

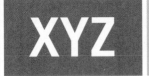

XYZ

xanthan (ZAN-thun) **gum**—a polysaccharide produced from bacteria; a thickener, emulsifier, and stabilizer.

X chromosome—sex chromosome; female.

xerosis (zee-ROH-sis)—dryness of the skin.

XXY chromosome phenotype—also known as Klinefelter's syndrome, when males have an extra X chromosome. The most common of sex disorders. Those who are affected often have female secondary sex characteristics such as wider hips, breasts, and female-patterned balding.

xylocaine (ZYE-loh-cayn)—*see* Lidocaine.

xyloglucan (ZYE-loh-gloo-kan)—an extract from plants; antiseptic in nature.

Y chromosome—sex chromosome; male.

yearly business objectives—part of the annual business plan which identifies the goals a business would like to attain during a given fiscal year.

yeast infection—viral infection caused by several unicellular organisms which reproduce by budding. Oral yeast infections are common in those with compromised immune systems.

yeasts—unicellular fungi.

yin and yang—concept originally devised by Fu Xi that describes the harmony between nature and its daily phenomenon.

zinc oxide—physical sunscreen which scatters light rather than absorbing or filtering it.

zosteriform—arranged along a nerve, as in shingles.

zygomatic major—muscle of the mouth which acts to purse the lips.